ೀೀೀೀೀೀೀೀೀೀೀೀೀೀ

More Than Just Veggies

Healthful, Conscious Eating in the 21st Century

ೀೀೀೀೀೀೀೀೀೀೀೀೀೀ

by Amy Erez
with help from Ofer Erez and Yo'el Erez

More Than Just Veggies
Healthful, Conscious Eating in the 21st Century
Copyright © Amy Erez 1999

Hands of Joy Press
c/o Health Etc.
P.O. Box 4999
Walnut Creek, Ca
94596

Cover photograph by Amy Erez

Library of Congress Cataloging-in-Publication Data
Erez, Amy, 1957 -
    More Than Just Veggies: Healthful, Conscious Eating
in the 21st Century/ Amy Erez
        p.   cm.
    Includes index

ISBN 0-7392-0478-5
Library of Congress Catalog Car Number: 99-96945

First Printing, 1999

Printed in the United States of America

Printed by Morris Publishing, Kearney, NE

All Rights Reserved. No part of this book may be reproduced in any form, electronic or otherwise, except for brief reviews, without the written permission of the author or publisher.

A portion of the proceeds from sales of this book will be donated to Mothers for Natural Law or other organizations which support the continuation of pure, organic food and the health of our planet.

ଛଡ଼ଛଡ଼ଛଡ଼ଛଡ଼

Dedicated to:

My mother, Irene Shirley Ehrenreich, whose love of cooking led me to discover that creativity can be found in the kitchen.

ଛଡ଼ଛଡ଼ଛଡ଼ଛଡ଼

Acknowledgments and Appreciations

Many heartfelt thanks to Ofer and Yo'el for their honesty and willingness to sample all of my experiments. Also to Rebecca, Eileen, Sherry and Ofer for their thoughtful, invaluable feedback. And most of all, great gratitude to *all* of my students who encouraged me to write this book for them. Without you it would have remained but a dream!

ଛଡ଼ଛଡ଼ଛଡ଼ଛଡ଼

Table of Contents

Preface 6

Chapter One: Eating for Health.................. 7

Chapter Two: Food as Sacred,
            Food as Medicine.................. 13

Chapter Three: What is Genetic Engineering?
            Why is it Harmful?............... 19

Chapter Four: Altering the Nature of Food
            and the Environment........... 24

Chapter Five: Follow Your Inner Knowledge.. 30

Chapter Six: Why Organic?....................... 37

  Introduction... 45

Appetizers, Sandwiches, Pizzas and Sauces... 47

Simply Salads.. 75

Scrumptious Soups................................ 91

Basic Beans... 111

Great Grains... 115

Casseroles and Other Stuff........................ 123

Pleasing Pastas.. 143

Tantalizing Tofu, Tempeh and TVP............. 155

A Thanksgiving Feast............................... 177

Delicious Desserts and Drinks.................... 187

Footnotes... 221

Recipe Index... 223

"I am not leaving home, I am not leaving home,
I am returning, I am returning.

I am not leaving home, I am not leaving home,
I am returning, I am returning.

Mountain, river and sea,
Living in me,
I am returning, I am returning.

Mountain, river and sea,
Living in me,
I am returning, I am returning."

Susan Osborn

Preface

In the beginning, science was an exploration of the world around us for the purpose of understanding the wonders that surrounded us daily. Somewhere along the way, this awe and wonder turned into a desire to be in complete control of the world and all of its systems. As the ego grew stronger, science became a forum for manipulation of the world rather than a place of worship. The larger the human ego becomes the further we go astray from our original intentions of discovery and understanding. We, as a species, are wandering further and further from the holy connections we have with all of nature as we yearn to perfect something that is already perfect. I became fully aware of the depth of the condition of our planet without really trying. I found this information plastered on the pages of the local newspapers and magazines that I read daily. I never needed to go searching in obscure journals for proof or the motivation to make changes in the way I live. I intend with this book to provide a glimpse into how valuable it is for us to return home to a world that has been created perfectly to support our every need instead of leaving this holy place in search of something more. I hope that you may find within these pages the inspiration you need to look inside yourself for the home that you have wandered so far to find. Our children's lives depend on it.

Chapter One

֍

Eating for Health

My Personal Journey: The Growing Years

When I was a teenager, I had a great desire to heal the planetary wounds that I saw around me. I looked to our government and political action at first and found it all so overwhelming that I removed myself from it completely for many years. I found so much pain in the world that it was easier for me to withdraw from it than to look for viable solutions. Instead, I discovered that I could look to myself for healing. I hoped that as I found my own health and peace that it would send ripples out into the world and cause a healing effect there as well.

My knowledge and understanding about food and its relationship to life on earth began as a search for my own health and well-being. As a young teen I found that a good way to squelch my sorrows was to feed my emptiness inside. So I continually fed myself to keep away the empty feeling. The only way I could get myself under control was to do a calorie counting diet which became an uncomfortable pattern of obsession about what I was putting into my mouth. It did help me lose weight though and for a few years things seemed ok.

In my years as a child and teen, I had numerous occasions when my body was pumped full of medications in order to create better health for my body. After three surgeries and an endless supply of antibiotics for adolescent acne, I was tortured for years by yeast infections, bladder infections and instructions from my doctor never to eat citrus again. My food intake was pretty pathetic.

Filled with sugar, preservatives, meat, dairy and frozen vegetables I didn't know that I was creating more symptoms by the way I was eating. It was the only way I knew to eat. When I went to college I realized that I could make my own choices about health care. I decided to ignore all of the advice and admonishments I had received and find a way to be truly healthy.

By this time I had learned to eat before I was hungry for fear that I would feel empty again and be in a place where there was no food. So I would overstuff myself, especially right before exercising, in order to give myself energy to do my exercises! I had no idea, as I continued to be overweight, even with regular vigorous exercise, that I was fat because I was so afraid of the emptiness inside of me!

I learned how to meditate as a young adult and I discovered, quite by accident, that I was learning how to fill myself up in a different way. I learned how to feel real hunger and that to feel hungry was a feeling of power and strength, not the weakness I always thought it would be. Without any intention of losing weight, I found that pounds simply melted off of me. As I meditated regularly, learned to use affirmations to change the way I thought of myself and my life and discovered how to love myself, I also had a new body in which to live. As the weeks went by, dear friends would not recognize me, and even my father did not know it was me twice within one hour! It was during this time that I came to understand that weight-loss was a spiritual experience not a physical or self-controlling one!

✿✿✿✿✿✿✿

"Meditation is not a goal but a process, a kind of awareness that is not alien to you, but is inherent in your nature. It is not something you have to try to do, but rather a process you must allow to happen, with as few preconceptions as possible. It is not someplace to go; it is a state of being."

Elson M. Haas, M.D.

✿✿✿✿✿✿✿

Lots of Experimentation

I experimented with myself time and time again. Vegetarianism done poorly was my first experience of attempting to eat healthily without actually doing so. As a college student, I and my friends would cook for huge potlucks of rich dishes like very cheesy Eggplant Parmesan and high-fat desserts like Trail Mix cookies filled with nuts and honey. We would eat to overfull for hours and then do it again the next weekend. During the week, quesadillas and chips and salsa were a staple. We thought we were eating in a healthy way, because our meals were vegetarian. The overabundance of cheese, breads, sweets, sauces and alcohol during those years was actually creating more health problems, instead of helping them as I had wished. I found that over time, I was somewhat hypoglycemic and unable to continue eating vegetarian because I was craving meats to balance the dairy and sweets in my diet. My understanding of this became a little clearer as I studied Eastern dietary ideas and I could see my own patterns. Although I continued to practice my meditation, I couldn't change the patterns that I had established in my body. This time I realized that I was physically sick.

Eventually, I discovered a wonderful book on macrobiotics (a dietary style based on the balancing of yin and yang foods, which includes meats and sugars at the ends of the spectrum). In my enthusiasm, I unintentionally became strictly macrobiotic in my eating habits and the experience I had years before was repeated. Without even trying, I slimmed down and had much more energy to live. This time, however, I also stopped my meat and sugar cravings and my acne problems virtually disappeared. As I looked at this experience more closely I tried to understand what had happened. Was it this strict way of eating that was having such a profound effect? Wasn't the meditation the important element in my weight? I was actually somewhat confused.

Quality Equals Taste and Health

At this time, I also started to learn organic gardening and to purchase more organic foods at the health food store. I found that not only was I spending less money for food, but I was eating more than ever and still losing weight! I was amazed. I had never experienced being able to eat my fill every day, three meals a day without feeling overstuffed, lethargic and gaining weight. I started to experiment with organic versus non-organic foods. I found that they also tasted much better. The fact that I was eating fewer sweets and no meats, made my food expenses go down. I also was enjoying the work in the garden and the vegetables that we grew helped to lower the food bill during the summer. I became aware that the choices I unconsciously made during different seasons related to the seasonal needs of my body. In winter and early spring, I eat green, leafy salads to balance the heavier warm foods that make up the major part of the meal (soups, casseroles, grains, stews). In the late spring/summer /early fall, I desire different types of vegetable salads and only use lettuce on sandwiches or not at all. This intuitive choice made me aware of the large variety of fresh vegetables and fruits available during summer versus winter and how much more nutritionally valuable they are to me than lettuce.

✿✿✿✿✿✿✿

"The seasons change; we change. When we move outside the laws of nature, or resist change, we encounter difficulty. If we learn to live within these laws we will know health as our friend."

Elson M. Haas, M.D

✿✿✿✿✿✿✿

All my life I had disliked water. During college I discovered a love of water from the mountains. I would drink water only when I was camping. I remembered this odd experience when I became macrobiotic and I began drinking bottled or purified water regularly. This was closer to my experience in the mountains! I understood that the additives in the city water were distasteful to me and for good reason. Now I could drink the water that I knew would bring me closer to health without adding more chemicals into my body at the same time. Slowly all of these different experiences helped me to realize that the purity of ingredients was important not only to taste but to my health too.

Another Step in Healing

As my life has moved onward, I have continued to be motivated in my self-discovery through my own pain. I have had physical ailments awaken to remind me that there is still more to learn. I began in my late thirties to experience horrible pains in my abdomen and sweats that would keep me awake at night. I had spent many years doing healing work with myself, including the dietary changes that I mentioned above. I was completely taken aback by these new symptoms when I was so healthy! After visiting my naturopath about this pain, she gave me a remedy to take and told me to stay away from any food allergens. The next morning after only one dose of this remedy, all of my aches and pains were completely gone! The next evening, I found myself craving roasted chicken that I saw at the store. I had some for lunch and munched on it again that evening. I awoke that night with the worst case of symptoms I had yet experienced. At that moment I realized that the chicken was an "allergen" I had not previously considered. I discovered that my symptoms were being caused by my intake of meat (I had not eaten pork or beef for years, but I still ate chicken, turkey and fish). At first, I was able to continue to eat fish, but after some time I also had a reaction to that. It turned out that I had "leaky gut syndrome" which had been caused so many years ago by the medications and foods that I had ingested as a youth. In my desire to ease my pain, I again became a vegetarian. This time I did it in a completely different way. It was my body rejecting meats, not my mind. I found that as long as I was getting enough protein through soy foods, that I could be meat-free without the discomforts that I had experienced earlier in life. Soy is a wonderful substitute for both meat and dairy. It provides the textures, tastes, cooking qualities, vitamins and minerals necessary for an enjoyable and diverse diet that is healthy.

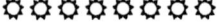

"You have a new car to start driving around-it's your body. Get it out of the garage, shine it up, and take it for a spin. You may even realize you have a third and fourth gear. If it appears to need a little tune-up, get it checked; but often just driving it will have it purring in no time. Remember to feed it lots of light, wholesome fuel this summer. Fresh fruits and vegetables, lots of water and juice, big salads, and some whole grains will give it the power it needs."

Elson M. Haas, M.D.

Chapter Two

❦

Food as Sacred, Food as Medicine

On Being Vegetarian

As I experienced my current vegetarian diet, I started to notice for the first time that I was actually feeling repelled by the idea of eating flesh. In the past I had proudly claimed that I was a vegetarian for health reasons not moral ones. Suddenly I was beginning to understand how my friends had felt when they said they couldn't even imagine eating meat again.

✿✿✿✿✿✿✿

"Faced with neatly packaged portions of meat or fish we no longer make the connection between the product and the animal that has been killed - unnecessarily for our sakes."
      Lucy Lidell et al., "The Sivananda Companion to Yoga"

✿✿✿✿✿✿✿

I heard somewhere the saying "a vegan is someone who won't eat anything that has eyes or a mother." I found myself thinking about this a lot. I was the mother of a young child myself. How would it feel to eat someone else's child? Or to have someone eat mine? It may seem a bit farfetched to you, but I found myself becoming more aware of the pain that animals go through during the process of being raised for butchering. Even the fish, though some are from the free-flowing ocean, are treated inhumanely during capture and slaughter. As the meat left my body I began to experience an internal connection to all of lie that I had not been aware of in the past. During my daily meditations, I could feel the energetic interdependence between myself and the natural world around me. Previously, I had felt that I could only experience this connection when I was out in nature. It was quite a surprise to feel this while sitting in my tiny suburban condominium! As this awareness deepened, I began to understand the agony of the animals who are raised for feeding humans. The Native American practice of contacting the soul of the animal and asking for forgiveness before slaughter made a lot more sense to me. If we are unable to do that with all of the food we eat, how can we be a part of nature as we were created to be? Gratitude is such an important part of living with our eyes and hearts open. Food used to be and still should be treated as a sacred part of life that provides us not only with nourishment, but also serves as a medicine for both body and soul.

For many years, sugar was seen as the big culprit. Researchers spent millions of dollars on developing synthetic sweeteners to sell to the public in place of natural sweeteners like sugarcane or honey. The proclaimed detriment of sugar was that it was laden with unwanted calories and caused cavities. Now, the public is again being cautioned about another food element that is the bad guy. Get rid of it and all your troubles will be over! Fat. Oooh, such an ugly word, fat. How ridiculous. For years now, the experts have been telling us to stop eating fat. Fat-free, low-fat, oil-free, on and on. Get rid of all the fat in your body, test your body for its fat content to determine how much you need to get rid of. Children are now being told that they will get fat if they eat foods containing fats! This is outrageous. For millions of years, people have been eating fats in a variety of forms and surviving quite well. What is different now?

The eating habits of human beings are different. We have

stopped eating in moderation and have become a society obsessed with satisfying our every whim and having to control our binges. Instead of eating meat when it is available through hunting practices which sometimes left us without meat for periods of time, we are eating meat three times a day. Meals used to be prepared around meat in a very different way than it is done in the modern world. Meat was the flavor in a pot of soup, not the main dish. The addition of spices, herbs, vegetables and water made the meal more nourishing, flavorful and plentiful. Drying of meats allowed them to be available in small amounts during times of lack, like during the winter months when hunting was at a minimum.

✿✿✿✿✿✿✿

"Animal flesh contains a high proportion of toxins (80% of food poisoning cases are caused by meat or meat products) and tends to cause disease. It also lacks vital vitamins and minerals and contains more protein than we need. In eating meat, we compelling our bodies to adapt to an unnatural diet, for which they are not designed. Our teeth and intestines are very different from those of carnivores - in fact, the anatomy and physiology of the fruit-eating primates is closer to our own."
     Lucy Lidell et al., "The Sivananda Companion to Yoga"

✿✿✿✿✿✿✿

  In some recent articles in the newspaper, I was shocked to find that there are more types of pollution than I ever thought could become a problem. It seems that there are some pig farms, in the Midwest that have such strong, noxious odors coming from the large amounts of manure there, that people are unable to sleep in neighboring houses. President Clinton has even gotten involved and has supported the idea of a law limiting this type of air pollution![1] It is amazing to me that things have gotten so bad. It sounds like a horrific science fiction story: "Humans die of asphyxiation from local pig farms!" This hasn't really happened, of course, but movement is going in that direction. Cows continue to overgraze the land, turning once fertile farm lands into useless patches of earth unable to support even the smallest blades of grass. Once this occurs, the trees and other natural plantlife in a region also die out, and we end up with a new desert. Instead of raising hazardously high amounts of animals why not feed starving people all the grain that we feed the animals? I know this is not a new idea. What I don't understand is why hasn't it been done? Most likely, it is because the meat and dairy industries have such huge lobbying power through the billions of dollars that they make each year from selling dead, poisoned animals for people to consume.

✿✿✿✿✿✿✿✿

"The meat, once it is broken down to be assimilated and rejected, gives energy but doesn't build good quality blood or tissue. The process is too fast, the need to eliminate too strong. Thus, what does not follow the natural building process is continually rejected. This is the body's attempt to burn away 'dead' matter. Fever results when toxins are not eliminated fast enough."

Naboru Muramoto

✿✿✿✿✿✿✿✿

In today's world, we are stuffing ourselves with foods that have the natural fats removed and have added caffeine or sugar (often synthetic) to create flavor so that the emptiness is at least palatable. Over and over I am baffled at the commercials I see for foods that promote and brag about low-fat nutrition but are flavored with chocolate or synthetic butter.

The current news is that low-fat may actually harm some people. "A low-fat diet may not benefit you if you: replace fats with sugary "fat-free" foods, ... cut too much good fat (such as olive oil, fish oil)," says USA Weekend's article "Low-fat isn't always best". The article goes on to say "Harvard researchers recently concluded that total fat intake does not determine heart disease risk....increasing intake of saturated animal fat boosted heart disease risk 17 percent." [2]

Another article tells us that butter is not the culprit we once thought it was, actually margarine is worse. "The study of more than 80,000 nurses by the Harvard School of Public Health and the Brigham and Women's Hospital, both in Boston, showed that the risk of suffering a heart attack was 53 percent higher among women who consumed the largest amounts of transfats than among those who consumed the smallest amounts. The greatest source of transfats in the American diet? Margarine."[3]

"A new study adds to growing evidence that eating monounsaturated fats - the kind found in olive and canola oils - may significantly reduce the risk of breast cancer."[4]
"As women enter menopause, their risk of heart disease skyrockets. One common recommendation - to drastically cut fat and eat more carbohydrates - is a bad idea , says Stanford's Gerald Reaven, M.D." "Reaven insists that a diet high in fat (45 percent of calories, mostly olive oil-type fat, not animal fat) and low in carbohydrates (40 percent of calories) reduces heart disease risk better than an overall low-fat diet." [5] Not so long ago the experts were telling us the opposite information.

✪✪✪✪✪✪✪

"Nowadays, processing foods removes much of their natural salts, and then, for flavor, manufacturers add more salt (white sugar too) to many of these foods. Almost all packaged and canned foods have some salt added to them. This chemical can create physical and psychological addiction just as sugar does, and it starts early, as many commercial baby foods have added salt. "

Elson M. Haas, M.D.

✪✪✪✪✪✪✪

"You have a new car to start driving around-it's your body. Get it out of the garage, shine it up, and take it for a spin. You may even realize you have a third and fourth gear. If it appears to need a little tune-up, get it checked; but often just driving it will have it purring in no time. Remember to feed it lots of light, wholesome fuel this summer. Fresh fruits and vegetables, lots of water and juice, big salads, and some whole grains will give it the power it needs."

Elson M. Haas, M.D.

✪✪✪✪✪✪✪

Chapter Three

❧

What is Genetic Engineering? Why is it harmful?

Not too long ago, I started hearing enthusiastic reports about a new tomato that would be on our shelves soon that would travel well from the farm, stay fresh for weeks, and be beautiful for purchasing at your neighborhood store. There were no comments about the nutritional value or what possible harm that could come from such a fruit. Only pure propaganda saying, "Look, here's another improvement we've made on nature for you to buy!" I started to look into this phenomenon in a casual way. I noticed more and more articles appearing in the news about this new product. I began to realize with horror the depth of the possibilities for harm that this seemingly wondrous new food could cause.

These foods I am referring to are genetically engineered or altered foods. They are in your grocery store right now. On the shelves and in your families' tummies, without you even knowing it. Restaurants are serving these foods also, and they do not even know it; therefore, neither do you. These foods have been manipulated by geneticists to provide a number of unnatural traits that these scientists and the companies they work for have deemed valuable to the consumer. And, more importantly, to their pocketbooks.

"What are you talking about?" you may be saying right now. I am talking about a new technology that has been used to alter permanently the food chain as nature created it. These scientists are splicing genes from different plant species, animals, insects,

viruses, and bacteria into the crops that are being grown for human consumption. The DNA of our foods has *already* been permanently altered and has not been tested for safety before being put on our shelves and into our stomachs. We are the guinea pigs in this experiment.

What are some of the traits being pursued by these companies? Improvement of food production, pesticidal and herbicidal reduction, increase of crop yields to feed the world. Rather than achieving these goals, however, the production of plants containing genes that resist insects in turn creates a plant that wards off beneficial insects as well. This reduces the plants' ability to pollinate and bear fruit. A recent example of this occurrence was reported in the United States from a finding that "the caterpillars of monarch butterflies were killed by pollen from a genetically engineered form of corn in a laboratory test. The corn was modified so that it would be resistant to the corn borer."[1] Monarch butterflies are a primary pollinator in a natural environment. Some of these same plants have been identified as pesticides by the EPA (Environmental Protection Agency) rather than vegetables for human consumption. How does this increase crop yields to feed the world?

As if this wasn't enough, the idea of using fewer pesticides on these crops actually works in reverse. The insects evolve into an insect with greater resistance to the genetically engineered crops. This creates the need for farmers to spray more often and use larger amounts of pesticides and herbicides to fight off the newer, stronger insects.

In fact, these same companies that are producing genetically engineered plants for pest-control are also genetically engineering plants that do not go to seed. A plant that does not grow to a place of forming seeds is a sterile plant. This means that these plants are unable to reproduce themselves into future generations. Farmers who use these infertile seeds to plant their fields are committed to purchasing new seeds from the company to plant next year's crops. The natural course of farming is to collect the seeds from the current crop and use them for planting in the next planting season. Plants that do not give seed are like people who have had their ability to form sperm and eggs removed. This is exactly what is beginning to be seen in the world today. The evidence strongly points to our polluted environment as the cause of this change.

The way that seeds travel freely on the wind has already infected the world of plants as we know it. The genetically altered seeds will blow outside of the field boundaries cross-pollinating with the surrounding weeds that are desperately being held at bay in order to grow the foods we need. The next generation of weeds will contain the same genes as the genetically altered crops, thus requiring more pesticides to kill the weeds.

The seeds on the wind will also create a need for using more poisons because these genetically altered plants are already being grown in farmers' fields without restrictions or supervision, the seeds from these plants are blowing to neighboring fields and cross-pollinating with the crops grown there. It is possible that even certified organic crops, carefully tended for years, have already been infected by these new gene-bearing seeds. This alteration of the DNA in our food sources cannot be reversed. This is not to be taken lightly. Look at the results of blindly jumping ahead and using chemical and nuclear products that now we discover are highly toxic and dangerous to human health and all of life on earth. These are infinitely difficult to clean up, but at least the earth may be able to heal from these mistakes with the help of human care and awareness. *This gene pollution, however, is permanent and is knitted quite effectively into the very fabric of life.*

There are many ways in which genetic engineering is dangerous to our health and the environment. The splicing of genes from sources that are not natural to the host plant provides a situation where we are uncertain what the resulting effects may be. Many people are allergic to a variety of foods, so even if the gene being spliced is from a natural source originally, it may cause allergic reactions in people eating the altered food. The allergen can be transferred from the original source to the altered food. This phenomenon has already been discovered during trials of soybeans that were genetically altered with brazil nuts[2]. This could be fatal to an unknowing person who ingested a supposedly non-allergenic food. In addition, many peoples in the world choose to follow religious traditions on dietary intake. For a kosher Jew, for example, to eat a vegetable with a pig gene spliced into it is breaking strict traditions established thousands of years ago. Vegetarians who wish to avoid the intake of flesh cannot avoid consumption of animal genes when eating strawberries or tomatoes with "anti-freeze" genes from Arctic fish[3].

Eventually, those who wish to choose what they eat for whatever reason, will be left with nothing to eat because there will be no way of knowing what foods are pure. In fact, the purity of food itself has already been compromised by the lack of regulation in this industry. One example of lack of regulation is the use of the bacterium *Bacillus thuringiensis* which has been used to change the makeup of a strain of cotton. Although cotton is not directly ingested by humans, there are nearby fields that can be infused with these genes through the seeds' wayward movement on the winds. The use of bacteria and viruses in genetic engineering has created a dangerous situation in the realm of medicine, as more and more antibiotics become less effective due to the constant bombardment of superbacteria into the human system from the foods we eat[4]. What are the true results of these genetically engineered foods? No one knows for sure, but here are some of the conclusions that renowned scientists the world over are making:

According to Mothers for Natural Law, a non-profit educational organization, "Dr. Fagan, internationally recognized molecular biologist and former genetic engineer states, 'We are living today in a very delicate time, one that is reminiscent of the birth of the nuclear era, when mankind stood at the threshold of a new technology. No one knew that nuclear power would bring us to the brink of annihilation or fill our planet with highly toxic radioactive waste. We were so excited by the power of a new discovery that we leapt ahead blindly, and without caution. Today the situation with genetic engineering is perhaps even more grave because this technology acts on the very blueprint of life itself.' Dr. Fagan goes on to say, "Genetic engineers can cut and splice genes very precisely in the test tube, but the process of putting those genes into a living organism is extremely imprecise, inaccurate, and uncontrolled. Such manipulations can cause mutations that damage the functioning of the natural genes of the organism. Once a gene is inserted into an organism, it can cause unanticipated side effects. Mutations and side effects can cause genetically engineered foods to contain toxins and allergens and to be reduced in nutritional value.' "[5]

    The profound realizations I had while reading the material in the previous paragraph was beyond any words I can find now. It sank *deep* into my soul. I know that should you pause now and reflect on what you have just read, your life will change as drastically as mine has. We are a planet of sentient beings who are playing God through the manipulation, sometimes fatal, of the genetic makeup of our already perfect and beautifully designed world. The final results of this experimentation is truly beyond our ability to predict as human beings for our knowledge of life on the planet we inhabit is woefully incomplete.

Chapter Four

✥

Altering the Nature of Food and the Environment

✿✿✿✿✿✿✿

"We are what we eat. This statement is true in more senses than one. Food is of course necessary for our physical well-being. But as well as this it also has a subtle effect on our minds, since the essence of food forms the mind."
    Lucy Lidell et al., "The Sivananda Companion to Yoga"

✿✿✿✿✿✿✿

    The lack of respect for life and for the natural order within all of life is absolutely appalling to me. An example of this lack of respect came into my awareness once again through my local newspaper. "Animal study shows no use for menopause"[1]. What a headline, huh? The amazing disrespect for women as a valuable portion of the human race struck me full in the face. On the one hand, the article reports that "Menopause is a midlife milestone that, in the eyes of some scientists, is as important a signature of the human species as a large brain and an opposable thumb."[2] Then, in the next breath, it states that these studies were done on baboons and lions in Africa and the conclusions were applied to women! What in the world do baboons and lions have to do with the lifecycles of women? In a recent video of Christiane Northrup, M.D., author of "Women's Bodies, Women's Wisdom", she stated that there is a hormone that is at elevated levels during the menstrual cycle that remains elevated after menopause.

Apparently this hormone has effects similar to endorphins which are widely known for their benefits as energy boosters and natural sources of a relaxing effect resulting in a meditative state. What I find fascinating about this statement is that clearly the lifecycles of women are significantly different than that of men. And has this also been studied in baboons and lions? Why didn't these researchers simply study women and their lifecycles if they wanted to learn about the purposes of menopause? This is such a blatant disrespect that it is embarrassing and horrifying that it still exists in this day of enlightenment!

This disrespect of women and their natural lifecycles as a valuable part of life is also manifest in other areas of life around us. When you look around you at the young girls growing up during this time, what do you see? I have for many years noticed a change of earlier physical maturation, with grade-schoolers looking as though they belong in junior or high school. Along with early menstruation, comes early pregnancy and more teens dropping out of school and society, burdening themselves, their families and the government. I believe an increase in the hormones ingested through our food is responsible for this change. The most current example of this is the hormone RBGH which is injected into cows in order to cause them to produce more milk. There is quite a flurry over whether this should be acknowledged on packaging so that we, the consumers can choose whether or not to ingest hormones into our bodies with our milk.

"After reviewing nearly 300 studies, the EPA (Environmental Protection Agency) concluded in 1997 that hormone-disrupting chemicals 'can lead to disturbing health effects in animals including cancer, sterility and developmental problems.' " [3] There was inconclusive evidence at that time that similar problems are being caused in humans by these pollutants (from pesticides, plastics and other industrial pollutants), but the EPA recommended more research of the potential risks, especially when concerning children. The same article reports "A recent study of 17,000 U.S. girls showed that 48 percent of black girls and 15 percent of white girls showed signs of puberty by age 8. ...some researchers worry that ingredients in some shampoos, dyes and detergents are absorbed through the skin and then scramble hormonal signals." [4]

✧✧✧✧✧✧✧

"On Eating Chicken
The way things are going it would be wise for man to return to a simpler and healthier way of eating. Animal food has in some degree been part of the traditional diet of many countries; however, the meat that is currently available is a great threat to mankind. A simple story can illustrate this fact:

An American boy came to see me about a problem he had. He could not understand why he had girl's breasts. When I inquired whether he had taken hormones in any form, he answered in the negative. I wondered what could have caused the breast growth until asked him if he had eaten much chicken in the past few years. This time he did not hesitate to confirm my suspicions as to how this growth had come about. He even informed me that girl's breasts in men are not uncommon in America. Before we parted he asked me whether he could have any children. He had been married for quite a few years and had no children. A doctor whom he had consulted told him that there was no hope of his ever fathering a child. I expressed hope that his sexual condition would return to normal if he could abstain from animal food and adopt a grain and vegetable diet. After all, in this world nothing is constant.

One year passed. Last summer I heard that his wife had become pregnant."

Naboru Muramoto

✧✧✧✧✧✧✧

On the opposite end of the spectrum, the competitive sports like gymnastics and ice skating are seeing younger and younger stars arriving. Due to the hormonal changes in a young girls body, these same stars are coerced into starving themselves, becoming anorexic or bulimic, taking drugs, overworking their young bodies and creating permanent damage to themselves through this inappropriate treatment. Some of them delay menstruation and breast development through painful ways, still others end up permanently damaging their female systems so that they are unable to conceive children when they want to.

A New Way of Defining Food as Medicine

One of the newest fads on the market now is a substance called sitostanol which is derived from pine trees. This substance is being added to foods to reduce cholesterol. The intention is for people who have high cholesterol to be able to lower it by the intake of these foods laced with sitostanol instead of medications. Amazingly, the article that gives me this information states opposing ideas. On the one hand it says "Scientists say medical studies show it (sitostanol) works much like a medicine...". [5] Then the article goes on to say "...you are going to be able to affect cholesterol levels, to lower them, in a greater number of patients without having to go to medications." [6] What do they think sitostanol is? It is extracted from its original plant source with the intention of changing physical symptoms in people with high cholesterol and they don't consider this a medicine? This is how the very first medicines were created. It is the way current medicines are manufactured in the herb and drug industries. I don't have anything against using medicine when it is necessary. What I object to is informing the public, many of whom don't know any better, that this food is not a medicine! In America, we have the weakness in our society of thinking that more is better.

What happens to the person with high cholesterol who gets a hold of these cholesterol-lowering products and eats them continuously, even after the cholesterol levels have normalized? Are these food products going to be prescribed by doctors and monitored by doctors or nutritionists to keep people from overdoing it?

✧✧✧✧✧✧✧

" A baby calf weighs about 130 pounds when born. He will weigh about 240 pounds one month later. By that time he is already walking around. This rapid growth rate requires quick development and...bone growth in order to meet the needs required by activity and weight. This is the reason why cow's milk contains so much more calcium than mother's milk.

On the other hand, human's milk contains phosphorous. This element is very important for brain growth and development. The human baby develops his brain first, while the animal develops his bone structure first. Therefore, milk for a human and that of an animal naturally should be different. Giving cow's milk to the human infant, without thinking about such an order of nature, is too simpleminded."
Naboru Muramoto

✧✧✧✧✧✧✧

By continuous poisoning of the body with nonorganic foods and synthetic medicines, we deaden our very cells to the natural knowledge contained within us. In turn, without that cellular knowledge being transmitted to the brain, the body is unable to communicate clear needs for the maintenance of health and vitality. As a result, we consult others about those aspects of ourselves that are easily communicated by a healthy body. The experts in our society have a specialized knowledge that offers us valuable information that is otherwise time-consuming or difficult for us to obtain for ourselves. The problem remains, however, that we learn to listen to the ideas and opinions of "experts" who have also lost touch with their natural knowing rather than consulting the vast knowledge that is stored in the depths of our own cellular makeup. Now that I have attained the intellectual knowledge of those surrounding me (through books, consultations, etc.), and am aware of the limitations of these sources, I am left with many questions: What am I to do? How can I get clarity about what is best for me? How can I figure it all out?

Chapter Five

❧

Follow Your Inner Knowledge

As a Holistic Health professional, I have had access to many people who were dealing with many of the same problems that I have had over the years. Instead of trying to convince people to change their diets (a very difficult thing to do) I decided to show them how tasty healthy food could really be; and so easy to prepare. So my husband, Ofer, and I offered cooking classes for our clients to come and cook macrobiotic recipes with us and feast on the results!

As we welcomed people into our home to experience the joys of truly living food, I discovered a passion inside myself that had been burning for many years. Over and over again, the results were the same, the amazement and joy that our students had when preparing and eating these living foods was tremendous. The difficulty, however, lay in creating a consistency in their lives. As much as they loved the foods they ate, it was difficult to bring this new knowledge into daily life; no matter how simple the recipes or easy to find the ingredients. The obstacle was deeper than that. The obstacle was in the very fabric of our lives: the people around us, commercials on TV, articles in the newspapers, words of advice from our doctors, old mental patterns we had received from our parents and their parents and their parents on down through the ages.

✿✿✿✿✿✿✿

"We must learn to heal ourselves, it is our right. It is unnecessary to depend on others, however qualified, to do it for us. There are many ways to get rid of a cold besides simplistically taking pills which 'work' for one day only. The cure must be complete. When we know how clogged our organs and arteries are, we have an insight into the extent of our freedom. If his body fluids do not run freely, how free can a man then be?"

Naboru Muramoto

✿✿✿✿✿✿✿

From birth we and our families are taught to give our personal knowledge and power over to the experts to determine our health or conditions of sickness. We are instructed from the first moment of pregnancy to submit ourselves to the sterile and sanitary testings and proddings of a medically-trained individual. We are taught that we do not know about our own bodies well enough to know for ourselves whether we are doing well or not. Pregnancy is a window of opportunity to reevaluate our relationship to our bodies and its needs. During this time, we are naturally sensitive to all of the changes occurring within us. It is actually our *job* to stay aware of what we sense and fulfill the needs we discover immediately (eating more or certain foods, sleeping more at varying times of day, etc.). By the time the baby comes we are well-indoctrinated into looking to others for information about our babies and ourselves. Our inability to achieve this shift in ourselves is a sign of the detrimental changes in our society in recent generations. The isolation of family members from each other and the community members around them results in a lack in the lives of children as to the natural cycles of life. Children are no longer exposed to the opportunity to witness to the miracles of pregnancy, birth and death.

The mother, who is most intimately in touch with her baby's needs: physically, spiritually and emotionally, is trained to listen instead to the doctor's instructions. Well-baby visits are instigated with the idea that this will keep the baby healthy by catching early any symptoms that may arise. The parents are also often taught to put the baby on a regular feeding and sleeping schedule, which does not support the natural rhythms of the child. This completely strips the parents of confidence in their innate wisdom or even the possibility of being aware enough to notice their baby's needs. Both parents, become well-trained to run to the doctor when any type of variation in the child's behavior or physical constitution arises.

✧✧✧✧✧✧✧✧

"No responsible doctor will ever prescribe a medicine before making sure his patient understands the importance of a healthy, balanced diet. We should not fool ourselves into thinking that disease is caused by an enemy without. We are responsible for our diseases, for disease often results from mistakes in our choice of food."

Naboru Muramoto

✧✧✧✧✧✧✧✧

In the meantime, the child is observing and taking in the brainwashing as well. The child, who views the parents as all-knowing and powerful, sees the parents defer completely to the medical personnel. From this observation, the child learns that the experts know best and are not to be defied or questioned, that the personal knowledge of the individual is worthless and that only those outside of us know what is happening in our bodies.

Well-baby visits are a great assistance to many uncertain parents; and yet, there is a pattern of turning away from self-knowledge and toward the distant knowledge of the expert. Imagine how different it would be if we all had the ability to know ourselves well enough to feel what we needed and when (whether it be food, hugs, medications or a good night's sleep).

I am not suggesting that we all have the valuable knowledge that well-trained and experienced medical professionals have. I am suggesting that we are born with an in-depth ability to know ourselves and our needs on all levels of our being through the simple connection that we inherently have with all of life. Without even being aware of it we absorb others' ideas and make them our own. We create patterns or habits that come originally from those outside sources.

✿✿✿✿✿✿✿

"Oriental medicine has always taught that food is the best medicine. That is probably why traditional Eastern doctors did not expect to be paid; they believed that nature was doing the job, not they. In fact, it is said that in the ancient Orient doctors' salaries were suspended if their patients became worse, the doctor himself being held responsible for all expenses. It was agreed that the doctor's job was to keep people well."

Naboru Muramoto

✿✿✿✿✿✿✿

Choose Foods from Internal Awareness

Instead of continuing to follow your old patterns, notice the ways in which you are acting or eating habitually. Examine the sources of these habits and decide which ones serve you now and which ones do not. Try creating your own ways without forming new habits. Habits are not helpful, even when they are supposedly good, because they require a mindlessness that actually disassociates us from ourselves and our needs within each moment. So to create a whole new relationship with food and your attitudes about eating requires a constant mindfulness about what your body is telling you it needs and when.

Learn how to listen to what the body's message is by following your dietary habits and observing the resulting internal experiences. How do I feel when I eat a certain food? Or at a certain time of day? What do I do when I am upset and it is time to eat? When it's not a normal mealtime? Do I eat differently during different seasons? Or around different people? What are the old attitudes I have about what food combinations are healthy or unhealthy?

What happens when this way is followed is that we find ourselves eating the way babies eat, when they are allowed to eat in a natural way. One day I may want a lot of orange foods, another day cooked, or perhaps raw foods, few solids and lots of liquids one day and the reverse the next. The pattern is not initially recognizable. But it is there. What happens is that we learn to eat as we live. With an ebb and flow that matches our internal experiences. This awareness of ourselves creates a whole new way of living in the world. Look at what your life patterns are right now. Are they stiff and predictable or are they fluid and changing? Is the fact that they are ever-changing actually a predictable pattern? Unpredictability is also an unbalanced way to live. The middle way is best. Moderation is the key, not strict adherence to rules or rebellion against them.

✧✧✧✧✧✧✧

"The fertile and stable Earth we know as our Mother not only gives us the food that we eat-the Earth is our support on which we stand and lay ourselves to rest: our womb and our tomb. Being earthy or grounded is having our roots in a solid base. The Earth, revolving around its axis to make a day, relates to the cycles in nature, in man and woman, and is central to all the other elements."
Elson M. Haas, M.D.

✧✧✧✧✧✧✧

    As the years go by and I look more deeply into the many manifestations of my relationship with food and my body, I find that it is a reflection of the planet and the health of humanity in general that I am experiencing. Through my meditations I can feel the intimate connection I have with all of life. When I am in tune with the rhythms of the earth, I eat according to my actual needs, whether they be mental, emotional, spiritual or physical. If I am doing a lot of creative activities (writing, planning classes, thinking, organizing new projects, experiencing the inspiration of deeper knowledge…) I eat more because I am hungry more often. My brain activity burns fuel, which in turn requires me to refuel. The amounts are not necessarily larger, but usually more frequent or of a particular type of food. For example, I often eat spaghetti with marinara when I am doing a lot of creating, it provides my body and mind with the right kind of fuel to keep me going in a balanced way. I don't need to analyze why, just simply honor the desire and observe my reactions to the food I take in.

    When I ignore my intimate connection to nature, as I learned to do as a child, I find great pain and sorrow manifests in my life. I get confused and move through life without purpose, health or direction. Life becomes dull and meaningless when I do not feel the rhythms of nature flowing through me. During the years that I have found and strengthened this natural connection, I have experienced greater health, joy and clarity in life. Decisions become more obvious and painless as I am able to determine more readily what direction my life is going. I can then follow along willingly instead of struggling against the tide, wondering where I am going and how to save myself.

My personal power is directly connected to my willingness to be a part of the natural world. When I am ignorant of that connection and do abusive or habit-forming activities, I am in physical discomfort, weakened by self-hate. When I allow the power I receive from being connected to nature flow readily through me, my body returns to its natural weight and fitness as dis-ease lifts. I am able to expand my energy out into the world around me instead of holding it encapsulated in my limited body. Human beings have a divine energy that is directly influenced by the health of the planet. The plants, animals, rocks, all have life within them. As the life is drained from the soil, it becomes sand, unable to provide the spark for new life or to sustain that which originally sprouted from its womb. We see the same condition occur in plants, animals and people and we identify it as aging. Aging is simply the seeping away of the life energy that courses through us, until we dry up, become brittle and blow away with the wind.

✧✧✧✧✧✧✧

"They [Oriental medicine practitioners] know that our bodies are inseparable from the soil that feeds us. The earth, the plants it produces, the animals and mankind are all interrelated."
Naboru Muramoto

✧✧✧✧✧✧✧

Chapter Six

❧

Why Organic?

As I read the newspaper and magazines each day, I see the headlines that say: "Report finds world gets richer, Earth gets sicker"[1], "Study: Airborne Pesticides a Real Risk"[2], "Inhaled Steroids May Stunt Growth"[3], "Pesticides and brain tumors in children"[4], "Children at risk from pesticides in food"[5], "Farms may have to follow pollution rules"[6], "Thousands leave homes during fire at fertilizer plant"[7], "Modern distribution systems seen as cause of food poisoning rise"[8], "Environmentalists seek pesticide control review"[9], "New rules on tainted fish start Thursday"[10], "Upgrades sought for food safety"[11], "EPA bans use of toxic herbicide Bromoxynil on genetically engineered cotton plants"[12], "Water safety puzzle: chlorine byproduct is found...at levels associated with elevated miscarriage risk, but is 'fundamentally safe' "[13]. It is truly frightening.

How can anyone consider water that has shown an association with miscarriage "fundamentally safe"?! How can anyone go to the store and feed their children foods that may be covered with cancer-causing pesticides, or grown from genetically engineered seed that was created by splicing genes from viruses, bacteria, insects and pigs! How can you feed your families and yourselves meats that come from animals who have been locked in the dark in inhumane conditions, force-fed, and pumped with antibiotics? Or animals that have been fed their own manure? How can people continue to put pesticides on their lawns and growing fields while knowing that the same chemicals run-off into the water system from which they are in turn using in their homes, and the oceans from which they catch the fish that is served for dinner?

✿✿✿✿✿✿✿✿

"No one can tell you how to fit those seemingly nonexistent hours into your own life, for the simple reason that it's your life. But I can tell you about some of the individuals I know who have managed to give priority to the kitchen, for whatever reasons and by whatever means, and about what has come of their choice.

Tragically, the turning point often comes when health - our own or that of someone we love - is threatened. Suddenly the games food advertisers play are no longer amusing. You find yourself angry now, seeing the damage they have done. Your priorities shift abruptly. And when you see that what you do in the kitchen might make the critical difference for someone you love, many of the subtler forms of resistance ("I'm being exploited," "This is tedious," or "But I cooked last night") lose their force. Life, we realize, is very short."
                              Laurel Robertson et al.," Laurel's Kitchen"

✿✿✿✿✿✿✿✿

My passion for organic foods has strengthened through the years as I have come to understand how profoundly eating organic food affects my own health and the health of the planet. For many years, I have done all of the token environmentally correct things: recycling my bottles, cans, plastic and newspapers, using cloth shopping bags, reusing paper ones, using soap products without chemicals, eating foods without preservatives, not buying Mitsubishi products and so on. What I have only recently understood is how the choices I make about the food I eat is also an environmental issue. It is actually an issue that is reflective of the earth's ability to survive. It is about the ability of human beings to survive. It is about not torturing anything that has life whether plant, animal or human. It is about respecting *all* living things including the soil and the waterways, and the air we breathe.

    Not too long ago, I was visiting with my sister at my home. We commented about how wonderful it was to have so many birds singing around us. She asked me, "Do you know why there aren't so many birds any more?" I explained to her that numerous changes in the environment resulted in fewer birds. The covering of animal habitats by concrete to create shopping areas, homes, and streets is one way. One of the most insidious is the use of chemical fertilizers and pesticides on private properties. The quest for the ever-green lawn and no bugs or animals in our suburban environment has created a sad loss of food supply and living areas for birds and small mammals. When I take walks with my son and husband in the mild summer evenings, we witness at some homes dead worms who had crawled out onto the sidewalks to die, a sure indication that there has been recent spraying in the lawn. As we poison our lawns to provide weedless greenery, the worms die taking away a vital source of food for the birds. The natural food chain becomes interrupted. As we discussed the possible reasons for the lack of birds, she was amazed to discover how far-reaching the effects of pollution really are.

    I see so clearly now how intimately connected all of life is. Begin with the fertilizing of a farmer's field with strong, cancer-causing manmade chemicals. First of all, the people applying the fertilizer are breathing in these toxic materials causing direct damage to their internal organs. A striking example of this is the use of chemicals such as DBCP, Chorpyrifos and Aldicarb. These chemicals have been shown to be lethal or damaging to humans in very small amounts and are used regularly for controlling worms and insects in commercially produced bananas. There are no safety devices provided for employees who experience problems of vomiting, dizziness, reproductive mutations and the loss of fingernails[14].

Last year, Governor Gary Locke proposed creating a law limiting the levels of heavy metals in fertilizers, which are now virtually unregulated. According to an investigation by the Seattle Times "...some heavy industries, such as steel and aluminum manufacturers, are recycling their toxic wastes into agricultural fertilizers usually without the knowledge of the farmers who buy them." [15] Dioxin, a known carcinogen, is among them.

When the rain falls, the runoff fills the streams and sinks deep into the earth to the waterways below. Water evaporates from the polluted fields and becomes acid rain into our lakes and reservoirs. Drinking water is extracted from these lakes and reservoirs.

According to the article, "What you can't see in drinking water can hurt you":
'There are many ways for drinking water to become contaminated:
• Chemicals from factories, refineries, buried storage tanks and landfills can migrate to underground or surface water supplies.
• Animal wastes and pesticides may be carried by rain runoff to streams and lakes or seep into aquifers.
• Human wastes may be discharged into water supplies that are also used for drinking.
• Some hazardous materials, such as radon and radium, occur naturally and can contaminate local supplies.
Even water-chlorination systems, designed to kill bacteria, can create problems." [16]

The chemicals move with the water through the streams to the lakes and local creeks. Children and adults play and fish in the creeks, rivers and lakes. The water flows onward carrying these dangerous chemicals to the ocean killing, poisoning and mutating the fish and other sea animals along the way. Those that don't die are caught by people who eat them or leave them to die because they are not worth any money.

These same chemicals are now in the food the people are eating. It is in turn creating subtle changes in the anatomy, physiology and immune system of those who have ingested them.

Over time the residues build up in our bodies and we have new allergies to both natural and synthetic products. Our systems are unable to flush out the harmful additives (dyes, antibiotics, hormones) that are received through the foods we eat, on top of the medications we use to try to become healthy again. These chemicals are hidden in products that we use regularly to create health and beauty in our bodies. "Dozens of synthetic chemicals found in our food, environment and everyday products have proven harmful to wildlife and lab animals. Now there's a new focus on whether they're putting people at risk, too, by playing havoc with hormones that control reproduction and development." [17]

In recent years, a number of studies have been done on the effects of estrogen-like chemicals used in making pesticides and plastics. The studies show that these chemicals "...foul up sex cycles in fish and other wildlife."[18] "Hormonal havoc has [also] previously been reported in alligators, birds, river otters, carp and other U.S. wildlife.... Hormones play the same vital sexual role in humans as they do in fish and other animals."[19] We have started having lowered sperm counts, miscarriages, deformed babies, allergies to our environment, incurable diseases and we find that not only the fish in the ocean, but also the birds eating the fish, the animals eating the birds and we ourselves are becoming slowly transformed into a different species on its way to becoming extinct.

Our lives as human beings on this planet are inextricably intertwined with the rest of life upon the earth. The way people abuse the earth and all of her resources is not only damaging the earth, but is also changing the way that life itself exists in our universe. The mindless depletion of our resources is permanently changing the way that life on earth develops. Soon we will no longer have the seemingly endless possibilities of supporting human life on the earth. Without clean oceans and waterways, clean air to breathe, rich topsoil, and organic, natural foods we will not be able to survive. As animals and plants become extinct, the soil turns to sand and life in the oceans drains away, we are being faced with the fact that the sources of life energy available for sustaining us are disappearing. We, too, are becoming an altered species pushing ourselves blindly toward extinction.

Every day we inhale dozens of chemicals with each breath, ingest dozens more with each bite of food, waste more trees that supply oxygen to live on, kill more life in the oceans through oil spills, pollute more of the earth's natural plant life through the winds that blow genetically engineered seeds into the neighboring organic farmland and blindly go our way expecting that nothing will harm us.

✥✥✥✥✥✥✥

"Harmony of spirit and matter is essential to bringing about a healing process affecting ourselves, our families, and eventually the whole earth. Our era, our lives, our planet, all certainly need a cleansing and refinement as well as a new balance of earth and spirit. As individuals, we can help bring about this cleansing by reducing our own intake of chemicals and other toxins; of synthesized foods; and of diets heavy in flesh, eggs, and milk products; and by replacing these with a lighter, more natural diet of cleansing fruits and vegetables, whole grains, nuts, beans, seeds and sprouts; and by drinking uncontaminated spring water. And being out in nature whenever possible replenishes our spirits as well."

Elson M. Haas, M.D.

✥✥✥✥✥✥✥

Let's think about what would happen if instead of chemicals, natural fertilizers were put in the farmer's fields. Using composted materials and manure as natural fertilizers helps us in many ways. First of all, the farmer isn't inhaling dangerous substances while doing his job. Secondly, by composting and using manure we are recycling waste products that would otherwise be sitting in landfills or building up to create massive amounts of toxic materials that would not decompose properly, filling the air and earth with more pollutants. The rains from overhead would not be filled with evaporated chemicals. The rainwater would create runoff that would support an enrichment of the soil further downstream and in the neighboring lakes. Instead of killing both beneficial and harmful insects, the beneficial ones would flourish. They in turn would bring down the population of the harmful insects.

Companion planting (planting varieties of plants together that help each other grow without pests) is another valuable part of organic gardening. Crop rotation on a regular basis also helps to keep the soil alive and free of pests. To continually plant the same acres and acres of one crop year after year depletes the soil's nutrients without giving it time or materials to enrich itself to support future life. With regular crop rotation and companion planting, the soil becomes enriched regularly without additives of manmade nutrients.

By eating organic food and using organic products for pest control, we support a chain reaction of healing the earth and all of life. This chain keeps our farm workers healthy, keeps the oceans clean, allows our children to play in grass that won't poison them, renews the topsoil keeping the earth alive, gives us fresh air to breathe, keeps the beaches clean to play on, assists the natural process of pest control through the support of helpful insects and bugs. Eating local, organic foods supports the small farmer and the local economy, which in turn reflects into the national and global economies, the welfare of all animal life and the disastrous trend toward huge companies creating financial monopolies and creating a larger gap between the rich and poor.

We say to ourselves "It's not my responsibility", "I'm doing everything I can." What *can* we do? Start to eat foods seasonally.

Be aware of where your food comes from and buy fresh organic, locally grown foods. Don't eat grapes in winter for example. They don't grow in winter and are being imported from other countries full of horrible pesticides. Support your local economy through the use of foods that come either from your own area or at least your own country.

✿✿✿✿✿✿✿

"Time was - and not long ago - if you wanted to live in such a way as to be warmly connected with other people, the world supported your efforts. Today that really is not true. If you want community, in any form, or family, or home, you just about have to invent it. Your version will be unique with you. But the first and all-important step is to dig in where you are and 'make a place'."
          Laurel Robertson et al.," Laurel's Kitchen"

✿✿✿✿✿✿✿

Introduction

All the ingredients in these recipes are organic. On rare occasion I am unable to find an ingredient in organic form or it is so outrageously expensive that I find it hard to spend the money. On these occasions, I look inside myself and ask, "Will this food, in the amounts I intend to use it, be harmful to me?" ,"Would the recipe be good without this ingredient?, "Is there a simple organic replacement?", "Have I been eating a lot of non-organic foods lately?" I look at any new patterns that are forming or old ones that are flaring up and consider skipping this food until another time. If nothing feels out of sorts, I consider that my attitude is all-important, and I can choose to eat a small amount of this food feeling safe that it will not harm me.

When expense is my main concern, I remind myself that the cost of these pricey foods will wither when more people are buying them. The reality of our society's economics being based on demand is one I can have some personal affect on by purchasing organic foods. I have found over the years that prices are going down, while quality is going up. I am willing to do my part to bring down prices and make healthy, life-giving foods available to more people and eventually everyone.

I use seasalt in my recipes because it is a natural source of salt including the minerals that are so good for us. Iodized salt is not only a processed food, but also often has additives to make it go farther like sugar or corn starch.

I have found that dairy is a large source of discomfort for me personally and has the tendency to create problems for many other people as well. In most cases I use non-dairy products like soymilk or rice milk and find that they work as very good dairy substitutes. These days you can find soy yogurt, sour cream, cream cheese, etc. in health food stores. For those of you who are also allergic to soy, the rice milk is a great alternative, although a little sweeter in flavor. As always, however, I counsel moderation and find that I enjoy using some dairy on occasion. So, judge for yourself and choose what is best for you.

These recipes are simply ideas to take off from. Make them your own by leaving out ingredients, adding spices, using unusual substitutes or adding your personal comfort foods and flavors. Most important of all is to experiment freely without judgment or the need for perfection. Have fun, feel the joy of creating something new and how wonderful it is that this creation also sustains you!

ช่ช่ช่ช่ช่ช่ช่ช่ช่

> **As I see myself, so shall I be.**

✧✧✧✧✧✧✧

"There is no possibility of one's becoming a yogi, O Arjuna, if one eats too much or eats too little, sleeps too much or does not sleep enough."
                                                    Bhagavad-Gita 6.16

✧✧✧✧✧✧✧

Appetizers, Sandwiches, Pizzas, and Sauces

Avocado Dip

Prep Time: 5 minutes

I created this delicious and simple dip when I was looking for something different to dip steamed artichokes in.

- 1 ripe avocado
- ¼ cup mayonnaise or soft tofu
- ¼ cup plain yogurt
- 1 tsp. lemon juice
- 1 tsp. *It's a Dilly* spice mix

1. Mash avocado with a fork.
2. Mix remaining ingredients into mashed avocado and stir until well blended and smooth.

Serving Size and suggestions: makes 1 cup of dip or dressing for salads, over roasted potatoes or vegetables (page 139) or as a great dip for artichokes.

Avocado-Miso Sandwich

Prep Time: 10 minutes

When my husband first made one of these sandwiches, I thought it sounded awful. It grew on me over time and is now a family favorite. My six year old loves it too!

  1 ripe avocado
  4 slices whole wheat bread
  1-2 Tbsp. or to taste white miso

1. Spread the miso lightly over one side of two of the bread slices.
2. Open the avocado and spread half onto each of the remaining bread slices.
3. Close the bread slices into a sandwich and eat!

Serving Size and suggestions: Serves 1-2 depending on your appetite. This is a great travel sandwich for picnics, car rides, etc. Tastes great with green olives, carrot sticks and apple pieces.

Layered Mexican Dip

Prep Time: 30 minutes

This delicious dip is great for potlucks or just a simple summer meal when the evening is too hot to fire up the stove.

15 oz. can refried pinto beans
8-10 oz. guacamole
½ cup grated soy cheddar cheese
2 Tbsp. chopped scallions or chives
15 oz. can refried black beans
8 oz. sour cream
8 oz. salsa
2 Tbsp. chopped black olives

Guacamole:
    2 ripe avocados
    2 Tbsp. salsa or more to taste
    1 Tbsp. fresh lemon juice

1. Prepare guacamole by mashing the avocados in a small bowl. Add lemon juice and salsa and mix well. Set aside.
2. Mix a tablespoon of salsa into the refried beans, one for pinto and one for the black beans. Smooth the pinto beans onto the bottom of a one quart casserole dish or your favorite bowl.

3. Add the black beans on top of the pintos.
4. Spread the guacamole onto the black beans and then the sour cream.
5. Pour the salsa gently onto the sour cream.
6. Sprinkle the cheese onto the sour cream and sprinkle scallions or chives and black olives on top.

Serving Size and suggestions: Serve with tortilla chips or for a light meal add corn on the cob and a green salad.

Stuffed Portabella Mushrooms

Prep Time: ½ hour
Cooking Time: 15-18 minutes

Stuffed mushrooms are a true delicacy. When I was a child, I couldn't get enough of them. Now we have exotic mushrooms to add to the flavors and possibilities! This recipe may seem high in fat, but don't forget that we are not counting calories here and even modern science says a little butter is good for you!

1 ½ Tbsp. butter
1 small yellow bell pepper, minced
1 stalk celery, minced
¼ cup cooking sherry
1 ½ Tbsp. olive oil
½ onion, minced
6 portabella stuffing mushrooms
½ cup bread crumbs
½ tsp. marjoram
4 Tbsp. grated soy parmesan
salt and pepper to taste

1. Preheat oven to 350°.
2. Remove stems from mushroom caps.
3. Melt 1 Tbsp. butter and 1 Tbsp. olive oil in non-stick sauté pan over med-hi heat.
4. Place mushroom caps in pan.
5. Sauté for 2-3 minutes on each side.

6. Meanwhile, mince stems, onion, bell pepper, and celery, and mix in a bowl.
7. Set aside sautéed mushroom caps.
8. Add ½ Tbsp. butter and ½ Tbsp. olive oil to the same sauté pan.
9. Add minced vegetables and spices.
10. Sauté over medium heat for 3-5 minutes.
11. Add sherry to vegetables; cooking over med-hi stirring constantly for 2-3 minutes until most of the wine is evaporated.
12. Return cooked vegetables to the bowl. Mix in bread crumbs and 2 Tbsp. cheese.
13. Put caps in baking pan. Fill with vegetable mix, lightly patting down to fill completely, allowing extra filling to spill over and cover bottom of baking pan.
14. Sprinkle with remaining 2 Tbsp. cheese.
15. Cover and bake for 15 minutes.
16. Remove cover and broil for 2 minutes or until cheese is melted.

Serving Size and suggestions: Makes 6 stuffed mushroom caps. Serve with Broccoli in Cheesy Sauce (page 179) and Black Bean Salad with Mint, Lime and Herbs (page 75).

Tofu-Stuffed Wontons

Prep Time: 30 minutes
Cooking Time: 20 minutes

I have always loved crab-stuffed wontons and didn't want to give them up when I became vegetarian. So I created a delicious alternative made with silken tofu - that wonderful ingredient that can be used for so many dishes! This recipe won an award from Delicious! Magazine's Recipe Contest in 1999.

12.5 oz. Mori-nu silken tofu, firm
1 Tbsp. granular garlic
1 Tbsp. grated gingerroot
24-26 wonton wrappers (1/2 - 12 oz pkg)
1 ½ - 2 cups Spectrum organic canola oil
2 scallions, finely chopped
2 tsp. fresh lemon juice

Honey Sweet and Sour Sauce:
¼ cup catsup
½ tsp. sesame oil
2 ½ Tbsp. rice or apple cider vinegar
2 tsp. cornstarch

1. Blend tofu to consistency of ricotta cheese.
2. Add other ingredients for wontons and mix well with a spoon.
3. Place wonton wrappers in small pile at the edge of a cutting board.

4. Have 2 - 9" plates ready for folded wontons.
5. Pour a little water into a finger bowl and place next to wrappers. Have filling set conveniently next to wrappers.
6. Place wrappers on the board until filled with small spaces in between wrappers.
7. Drop a teaspoonful of filling onto the center of each wrapper.
8. Dip a fingertip into the water and wet one tip of a wrapper. Lift the opposite tip to the wet one and squeeze together until stuck. Do the same with the remaining tips and repeat with all the wrappers on the board.
9. Set finished wontons aside on a plate.
10. Heat about 1 ½ cups of oil in a wok until hot; keep at med-hi or hi heat while cooking wontons.
11. Add 4-6 wontons at a time, depending on the size of your wok.
12. Cook on both sides until golden brown. Make sure wontons do not stick together when cooking. Be very careful turning wontons because the oil will splatter.
13. Drain wontons on paper towels when removed from oil.
14. Prepare Honey Sweet and Sour Sauce by blending all ingredients thoroughly and warming over low heat until thick, stirring regularly to avoid sticking and burning.

Serving Size and suggestions: Makes 24-26 wontons. Serve as an appetizer or with a stir fry and rice.

Grilled Salat Tuna-Cheese Sandwich

Prep Time: ½ hour

Here's a great summer sandwich full of protein and dairy-free.

Salat Tuna:
  6 oz. tongol or albacore tuna in oil or water
  1 tsp. dijon mustard
  (if using tuna in water add 1 Tbsp. olive oil)
  1 Tbsp. tahini
  1 tsp. barley miso

12 slices whole wheat, 7-grain or 9-grain bread
6 slices American or Cheddar-style soy cheese
6 Tbsp. butter or margarine (for dairy-free)
1 medium tomato, sliced, optional

1. Fix Salat Tuna. If using tuna with oil, pour oil into salad. If using tuna in water, add olive oil.
2. Use ½ Tbsp. butter or margarine on each bread slice.
3. Spread tuna on unbuttered side of one bread per sandwich.
4. Place unwrapped cheese slice onto tuna. If desired, add a slice of tomato.
5. Place open sandwich in non-stick pan or skillet. Cover with another slice, keeping buttered side up.

6. Repeat #3-5 for as many sandwiches as you can fit in your skillet.
7. Grill over low heat about 2-3 minutes per side, allowing cheese to warm and outside to become golden brown.
8. Serve immediately or cool in refrigerator before serving.

Serving Size and suggestions: Makes 6 sandwiches. Serve with Barbecued Baked Beans (page 113) and Colorful Coleslaw (page 79).

Open-faced Mushroom Sandwich

Prep Time: 30 minutes
Cooking Time: 5 minutes

I keep hearing around town of these restaurants offering mushroom sandwiches. I haven't tried one yet, but it sounded so good and I love mushrooms sooo much that I decided to create one of my own. This is the simple and elegant result.

   4 large portabella mushrooms
   ½ lb. shiitake mushrooms
   1 loaf whole wheat sourdough bread
   1 Tbsp. balsamic vinegar, optional
   2 tsp. soy sauce
    ¼ cup pesto (page 69 or 70), or more to taste
   seasalt and pepper to taste
   ½ cup red wine
   ½ - ¾ cup grated asiago cheese or smoked soy monterey jack cheese
   4 tomatoes, sliced
   4 Tbsp. olive oil
   2 Tbsp. butter
   2 cloves garlic, minced

1. Remove stems from mushrooms and slice the mushroom caps. Use mushroom stems to make a broth for another time.

2. Melt butter with olive oil in large skillet over medium heat.
3. Add minced garlic and mushrooms for sautéing.
4. When mushrooms are getting soft and are a rich brown in color, add the wine.
5. Simmer for 2 minutes.
6. Add the soy sauce and cook for 3 minutes or so until the wine is almost completely evaporated.
7. Remove the mushrooms from the heat.
8. Cut open the loaf of bread as for a sandwich.
9. Spread pesto liberally on the bread.
10. Drizzle the balsamic vinegar into the mushrooms if desired.
11. Spread the mushrooms on the bread.
12. Place the sliced tomatoes over the mushrooms, and sprinkle lightly with salt and pepper.
13. Spread cheese over tomatoes.
14. Broil sandwich for 3 minutes or until cheese is melted and edges of bread are lightly browned.

Serving Size and suggestions: Serves 6 when served with a salad or grain on the side.

Variations: Try different cheeses, wild and domestic mushroom combinations, flavored breads instead of plain sourdough would be great if you want to leave off the pesto.

Pita with Roasted Vegetables

Prep Time: 1 hour to prepare vegetables,
30 minutes to prepare everything else

I was planning a trip to the beach and needed something yummy to bring. In looking through the frig I found plenty of veggies to roast and some leftover pita bread. So I created a spontaneous new pita sandwich! Here it is for you.

Roasted winter vegetables (page 139)
¼ - ½ lb. Bulgarian feta cheese
1 pkg. Organic pita bread
1 pint cherry 100 and yellow pear tomatoes
Tahina (page 71)

1. Prepare the roasted vegetables according to the recipe on page   . These may be prepared a day ahead and refrigerated overnight if necessary.
2. Wash tomatoes and remove stems.
3. Prepare tahini.
4. Slice pitas across so that they open easily into a pocket for filling
5. Serve all items in a buffet-style arrangement for serve yourself eating.
6. Prepare sandwiches by filling pita pocket with roasted vegetables, tahini, feta and tomatoes on top. Delicious!

Serving Size and suggestions: 12 pockets serves six hungry people. Excellent with fresh fruit and Honey Lemonade (page 217) for a fun summer picnic.

Pesto Pizza

Prep Time: 15 minutes
Cooking Time: 8 minutes

There are thousands of great recipes for pizza dough out there and also some great ready-made ones at your local store. So I have not included a recipe for pizza dough here. Pick your favorite crust and add these delicious toppings for a special treat! The cooking time here is based on a ready-made crust.

½ yellow summer squash, in small pieces
1 onion, chopped
½ zucchini, in small pieces
2 tomatoes, chopped
1 6-8 oz. jar marinated artichoke hearts
1 cup sliced mushrooms
¼ - ½ cup pesto, page 69 or 70
salt and pepper
1 Tbsp. olive oil
1 cup soy mozzarella, grated or more to taste
¼ - ½ cup soy parmesan, grated
your favorite crust

1. Sauté onion, mushrooms, zucchini and yellow squash in olive oil over medium heat until onion is translucent and vegetables are cooked but not limp.
2. Sprinkle vegetables with salt and pepper.
3. Spread pesto on pizza dough or crust.
4. Drain marinated artichoke hearts.

5. Add artichokes and tomatoes to sautéed vegetables.
6. Mix well.
7. Spread vegetables on pesto-topped pizza crust.
8. Top with shredded mozzarella and parmesan.
9. Broil until cheese is melted and slightly browned on top, 5 - 8 minutes.

Serving Size and suggestions: A 12" pizza can serve 4 easily, especially if it is served with a crispy green salad. Leftover veggies make a great filling for quiche, page

Variations: Add sliced green olives, vary summer squash types, grate instead of cut squash. Be creative!

Yummy Summer Sandwich Pizza

Prep Time: 15 minutes
Cooking Time: 5 minutes

This sandwich was created one night when I was going to make pizza and my yeast was moldy. Instead I used the same toppings on sourdough bread. Even easier and just as tasty! This sandwich freezes well. Make sure to reheat it in an oven, not a microwave, as the bread gets too chewy otherwise.

1 loaf french sourdough bread
2 medium tomatoes, sliced
¼ lb. mushrooms, sliced
1 small zucchini, cut in pieces
1 small peter pan squash, cut in pieces
2 Tbsp. olive oil
12 pimento stuffed green olives, sliced
1 small onion, chopped
½ cup pesto
½ lb. soy mozzarella, sliced
3 Tbsp. asiago, grated

1. Prepare vegetables.
2. Sauté all vegetables, except tomatoes and olives, in olive oil.
3. While vegetables are cooking, slice open bread.
4. Peel out inner layer of soft bread, leaving some to cover inner crust.

5. Place bread on baking sheet.
6. Spread half of pesto on each bread half.
7. Add olives to sautéed vegetables.
8. Mix well and spread onto bread halves until full.
9. Make sure vegetables are level with crust edge for a flat surface to place the tomatoes on.
10. Add tomatoes, mozzarella and asiago.
11. Broil until cheese is melted.

Serving Size and suggestions: Serves 4-6, depending on appetite. Delicious with a green salad.

Variations: Use any combination of vegetables that you like or make it more like a regular pizza by using vegetarian-style pepperoni slices instead of the main vegetables and tomato sauce instead of pesto.

Mushroom and Onion Marinara

Prep Time: 15 minutes
Cooking Time: at least 1 hour

This is a simple sauce using canned tomatoes and paste, with your own herbs for flavor. I love making fresh tomato sauce in the summer for this, but for most people that is more hassle than enjoyment. If you have fresh sauce, add fresh peeled and cut tomatoes instead of canned.

28 oz. can peeled tomatoes
6 oz. can tomato paste (sometimes I like to use the Italian-seasoned paste I find in the store)
6 oz. button mushrooms, sliced
1 tsp. dried thyme
½ tsp. dried marjoram or sage
2 tsp. dried sweet basil
2 tsp. dried oregano
1 medium onion, chopped
2 medium cloves garlic, minced
2 Tbsp. olive oil

1. Blend ¾ of the can of tomatoes, leaving some tomatoes in pieces for a chunky sauce.
2. Sauté the onion and garlic in olive oil for 2 minutes over medium-low heat.
3. Add mushrooms to onion and garlic and sauté for 2 minutes or until mushrooms are lightly cooked. Do not overcook mushrooms, they become mushy.

4. Add blended tomatoes, tomato paste, and spices to sautéed vegetables.
5. Bring sauce to a simmer over medium-high heat, reduce to simmer and cook for 1 hour without a lid to let water from tomatoes evaporate.
6. If sauce is thicker than you like, add a dash of red wine or water and cook to desired consistency.

Serving Size and suggestions: Makes about 20 oz. of sauce.

Variations: Add sliced black and green olives for a change.

Pesto

Prep Time: 15 minutes

Pesto is a flexible and fun food that can be used on sandwiches, pastas, salads, pizza, and veggies. Be creative and enjoy. It is delightfully healthy, too!

- 1 bunch fresh basil
- 1 bunch Italian parsley
- 3 small-medium garlic cloves
- ½ -3/4 cup pine nuts
- 1 cup olive oil, more or less to taste
- ¼ - ½ cup soy parmesan or asiago cheese

1. Wash parsley and basil thoroughly, removing stems.
2. In food processor, place parsley and basil.
3. Pour olive oil over herbs, add nuts, garlic and cheese.
4. Blend thoroughly, making sure that mixture is smooth and moist when done. Add olive oil as necessary to blend easily.

Serving Size and suggestions: Makes about 2 cups depending on size of herb bunches. I like to freeze pesto in old baby jars or whatever small jars you have around to enjoy all winter long.

Variations: Use different nuts: walnuts, pistachios, cashews; whatever strikes your fancy! They all add a unique flavor. Also, lemon basil is a must for a special summer treat instead of regular basil.

Basil-Walnut Pesto

Prep Time: 10 minutes
Cooking Time: 20 minutes

Pesto is such a treat in the summer! We love it so much and it is so easy to make that we make huge amounts and freeze them in old baby jars to continue enjoying into the winter. Growing unusual varieties is also fun for a different flavor (lemon, anise, dwarf etc.).

1 large bunch fresh basil
¼ - ½ cup parmesan or asiago cheese, soy alternatives work well too
2 medium garlic cloves, minced
½ cup olive oil
¼ cup walnut pieces

1. Wash basil thoroughly. Take leaves off the stems.
2. Place all the ingredients into a blender, food processor or use a cuisinart.
3. Mix thoroughly until smooth and creamy. This takes some doing and may require added olive oil to make it easier to do.
4. Add cheese, walnuts or garlic to adjust flavor to fit your personal tastes.

Serving Size and suggestions: Makes about 8 oz.

Tahina

Prep Time: 5 minutes

This delicious Middle-Eastern sauce is used liberally in Israel, the country of my husband's birth. This is the way he taught me to make it. Our son eats this like candy. It's great for picnics, school lunches and snacks as well as the main course for a refreshing summer meal.

½ cup Tahini (sesame butter)
2 ½ Tbsp. fresh lemon juice
6 Tbsp. water
1 Tbsp. olive oil
½ tsp. garlic powder
sprinkle paprika

1. Pour the tahini into an attractive serving bowl.
2. Add the water and lemon juice. Mix thoroughly.
3. Add garlic powder and stir well.
4. Spread sauce evenly in bowl.
5. Drizzle olive oil on top in a nice design.
6. Sprinkle with paprika.
7. Serve.

Serving Size and suggestions: Serve with whole wheat pita bread for dipping, cracked green and kalamata olives, pickles, cubes of feta cheese, sliced tomatoes, avocado slices and a tall glass of Honey Lemonade (page 217) for a simple meal; or serve over Tempelafel Patties (page 168) in pita with Israeli Cut Salad (page 85).

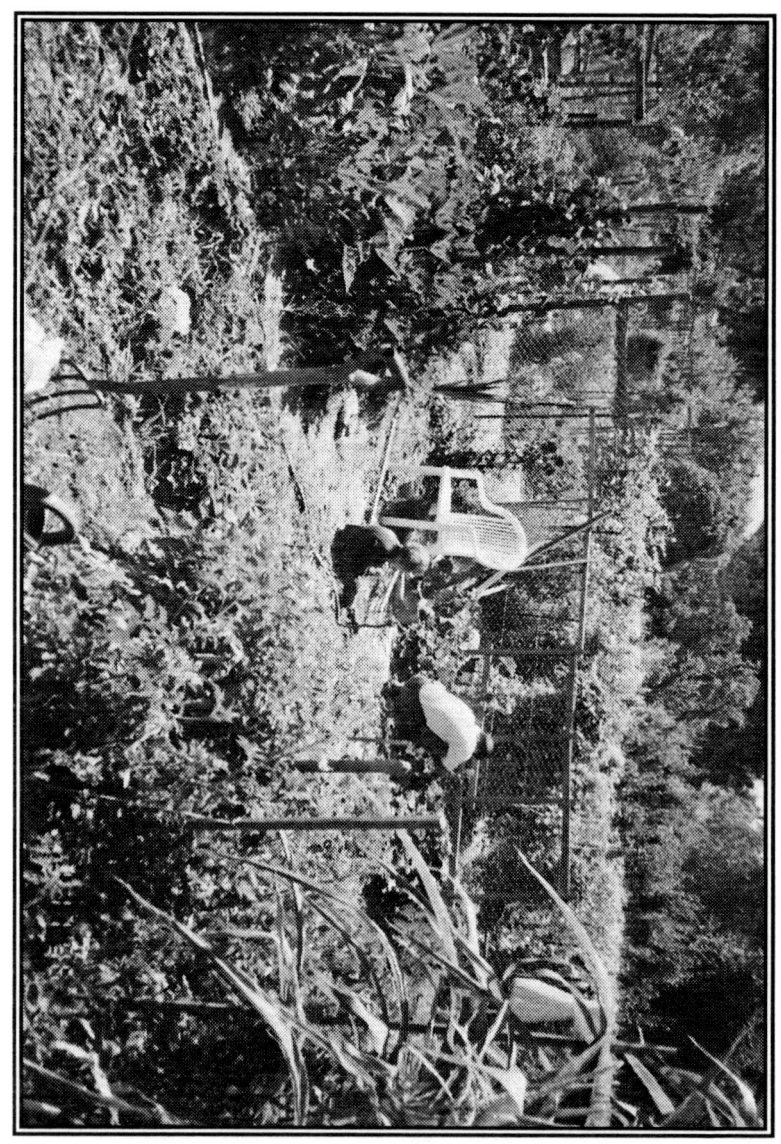

✧✧✧✧✧✧✧

"By eating properly we strengthen ourselves, body and mind, so that in the event of disease we do not have to panic and put ourselves at the mercy of the first curative technique that is presented to us."

Naboru Muramoto

✧✧✧✧✧✧✧

Simply Salads

Black Bean Salad with Mint, Lime and Herbs

Prep Time: 15 minutes
Refrigerate 2-3 hours

Ready for an unusual salad with enticing flavors reminiscent of exotic worlds? Here's a simple escape to a different land. Have fun!

15 oz. black beans
2 Tbsp. garlic oil
1 medium green zucchini, cubed
1 medium Japanese eggplant
1 medium yellow squash, cubed
3 Tbsp. lime juice
2 Tbsp. minced mint
2 Tbsp. minced Italian parsley or cilantro
1 small clove garlic, minced
3 Tbsp. feta, crumbled
dash white pepper and seasalt
1 Tbsp. olive oil

1. Wash eggplant, slice in half lengthwise and then slice thinly. Spread evenly on baking sheet.
2. Mix eggplant with garlic oil and roast at 350° for 10 minutes, stir occasionally to keep from sticking.
3. Prepare squashes and blanche in 2 cups of boiling water for 2-3 minutes.
4. Drain and rinse black beans.

5. Drain and cool squash.
6. Mix all ingredients, except feta. Refrigerate for 2-3 hours.
7. Crumble feta on top of salad before serving.

Serving Size and suggestions: Serves 4.

Black Bean, Corn and Tomato Salad

Prep Time: 15 - 20 minutes
Cooking Time: Chill one hour before serving

This is a simple and delicious summer salad. Best in the heat of summer when the foods are garden-fresh and easy to prepare with little or no cooking. I use canned beans and dried herbs for quick and easy cooking, but if you prefer fresh beans and herbs that's great!

1 cup yellow and red cherry tomatoes
1 15 oz. can black beans, drained and rinsed
1 scallion, minced
1 cob corn, steamed and cut off cob
Dressing:
1/8 tsp. Chili powder
¼ tsp. Dried basil
1/8 cup canola oil
1 Tbsp. Red wine vinegar
dash salt and pepper
¼ tsp. Dried parsley

1. Husk corn and put on to steam for 10 to 15 minutes or until easy to puncture with a fork. Do not overcook. Corn should be crisp and juicy.
2. While corn is steaming, wash tomatoes and slice in half. Put in salad bowl.
3. Drain and rinse black beans. Add to tomatoes.
4. Mince onion and add to salad bowl.

5. When corn is ready, hold at end and slice corn off cob into salad bowl.
6. Mix dressing ingredients in blender or with cuisinart.
7. Pour over salad and mix well.
8. Chill for one hour.

Serving Size and suggestions: Serves 6 when used as a side dish salad. Excellent with hearty bread or Bulgur Pilaf (page 117) and Baked Tofu (page 163). Also good with Tempelafel Patties (page 168) for a lovely summer supper.

Colorful Coleslaw

Prep Time: 30 minutes

This is a wonderful salad for summertime picnics or just hot days that defy cooking. The seeds and tahini give it a slightly unusual flavor that will meet the most discriminating tastes.

½ head green cabbage, shredded
2 medium carrots, shredded
½ red pepper, sliced thinly
½ head red cabbage, shredded
½ green pepper, sliced thinly
1 cup golden raisins
½ cup sunflower or sesame seeds, toasted
1 cup snow peas, blanched

Dressing:
½ - ¾ cup plain yogurt
2 Tbsp. canola oil
½ cup soymilk
2 Tbsp. lemon juice
1 Tbsp. tahini
½ Tbsp. honey
seasalt and white pepper to taste

1. Prepare vegetables and mix in a large bowl.
2. Blend dressing ingredients well.

3. Pour dressing over salad. Mix thoroughly and chill for at least 2 hours, stirring occasionally to make sure all ingredients get well marinated.

Serving Size and suggestions: Serves 8.

ð•ð•ð•ð•ð•ð•ð•ð•ð•

Cool Beet Salad

Prep Time: 30 minutes plus chilling time.

I was looking for a beet salad recipe one day and couldn't find what I had in mind. So I created this one!

  3 medium red beets, sliced
  1 Tbsp. apple cider vinegar
  ¾ cup plain yogurt
  1 Tbsp. honey
  1 Tbsp. fresh mint, chopped finely

1. Steam sliced beets until tender.
2. Whisk yogurt, honey and vinegar in a bowl.
3. Chop the mint.
4. Add the cooked beets to the sauce and add the mint. Mix thoroughly.
5. Chill for two hours.

Serving Size and suggestions: Serves 6 as a side dish. Great with steamed corn on the cob, Barbecued Baked Beans (page 113) and Baked Tofu (page 163).

Fresh Peas with Edamame and Herbs

Prep Time: 15 minutes
Refrigerate for 2 hours

I was preparing a salad with fresh peas from the Farmer's Market and discovered that I didn't have enough peas. So I grabbed some shelled edamame (green soy beans) from the freezer to add. It turned out delicious!

- ½ c. fresh peas, shelled
- ½ c. edamame, shelled, fresh or frozen
- 1 c. corn, fresh or frozen
- ½ c. small cherry tomatoes
- ½ c. yellow pear tomatoes
- 2 Tbsp. red wine vinegar
- 1 Tbsp. lemon basil, minced
- 2 Tbsp. Italian parsley, minced
- 2 Tbsp. olive oil
- 1 Tbsp. mint, minced
- 1 scallion, chopped

1. Blanche the peas, edamame and corn in boiling water for five minutes.
2. Meanwhile, wash and mince the herbs.
3. Chop the scallions and wash the tomatoes.
4. Drain the blanched vegetables.
5. Mix all the ingredients well.
6. Chill for 2 hours, stir well before serving.

Serving Size and suggestions: Serves 4.

Green Bean Salad

Prep Time: 25 minutes
Cooking Time: chill 2-3 hours

If you like three bean salad, you'll love this! A fresh and simple salad for summer. You can replace the canned beans with freshly cooked ones if you like.

2 cups fresh green beans, washed and broken into bite-sized pieces
1 cup sweet white corn, fresh off the cob or frozen
15 oz. can kidney beans, rinsed and drained
2 scallions, chopped
2 Tbsp. red wine vinegar
2 Tbsp. olive oil
1 Tbsp. honey
salt and pepper to taste

1. Boil 4 cups water in a large pot.
2. Pour green beans and corn into boiling water and blanch for 2-5 minutes or until beans become a bright green.
3. While vegetables are cooking, drain and rinse kidney beans in colander. Pour into serving bowl.
4. Drain vegetables into colander.
5. Add blanched vegetables to kidney beans.
6. Add scallions, oil and vinegar, salt and pepper.
7. Drizzle with honey and mix thoroughly.
8. Chill for 2-3 hours or until well chilled. Stir occasionally during chilling time.

Serving Size and suggestions: Serves 4. Excellent with Yummy Summer Sandwich Pizza (page 65) and Honey Lemonade (page 217) for a simple and delicious summer meal.

Variations: Add a variety of vegetables: garbanzo beans, black beans, cherry tomatoes, chopped red pepper, etc. Just be sure to keep the same ratios as the salad grows (adding oil, vinegar and honey) or do replacements so it is essentially the same amount.

Salat Tuna

Prep Time: 10 minutes

Not every member of my household is a vegetarian, and probably not in yours either. So I have included a couple of fish recipes for you and your family to enjoy as well. This one was a creation of my husband, Ofer, who has an eye for the unusual. This recipe is a great picnic dish. I have taken it on outings a lot with my son and his friends. Every time I pull it out they eat it up in a flash!

- 1 6 oz. can dolphin-safe tuna in oil
- 1 tsp. dijon mustard
- 2 Tbsp. tahini
- 1 tsp. miso, red or white to your taste

1. Mix all ingredients, including the oil from the tuna can. Stir well and serve.

Serving Size and suggestions: Makes two sandwiches or a great dip with stone-ground crackers for dipping.

Israeli Cut Salad

Prep Time: 15 minutes

Here's another extremely simple and delicious dish that is inspired by Ofer's Middle-Eastern background.

1 medium avocado
1 large tomato
1 medium English cucumber
2 scallions, chopped
15 pimento-stuffed green olives
1-2 Tbsp. olive oil
1-2 Tbsp. red wine vinegar
seasalt and black pepper to taste
1/8 - 1/4 lb. Bulgarian feta cheese

1. Cut tomato, avocado and cucumber into small pieces and place in a medium-sized bowl.
2. Add chopped scallions.
3. Slice and add olives.
4. Add crumbled feta cheese.
5. Sprinkle gently with olive oil and red wine vinegar. Add seasalt and pepper to taste.
6. Mix gently until vegetables are well covered.
7. Refrigerate until serving time or serve immediately.

Serving Size and suggestions: Serves 4. Excellent with Tempelafel Patties (page 168), Tahina (page 71) and pitas.

Variations: Try different types of olives, feta cheese, or tomatoes. Add a dash of freshly chopped basil or a squeeze of fresh lemon.

Sliced Tomatoes with Lemon-Basil Miso Dressing

Prep Time: 20 minutes
Refrigerate 2-3 hours

A light and flavorful salad with fresh garden tomatoes and herbs. This dish has an Asian flavor from the rice vinegar and miso. The first time I made this dish, my son asked me three times what was in it because he liked it so much.

1 ½ - 2 c. sliced roma tomatoes
1 Tbsp. lemon-basil
¼ c. diced red onion
¼ -1/2 tsp. each salt and pepper

Dressing:
1 Tbsp. canola oil
1 Tbsp. rice vinegar
1 tsp. white miso
1 tsp, brown sugar

1. Slice tomatoes and put in medium-sized bowl.
2. Add diced onions.
3. Mix dressing and pour over vegetables. Mix well.
4. Add salt and pepper and lemon basil. Mix well.
5. Refrigerate for 2-3 hours before serving.

Serving Size and suggestions: Makes about 4 servings.

✧✧✧✧✧✧✧

"Miso is an alkalinizing food and its fermentation assists the body's digestion and metabolism. In Japan it is also said to improve one's resistance to illness. For those who wish to strengthen their systems, miso can be used daily as a broth, as it is said to be a good tonic. A teaspoon to a cup of boiling water is mixed. Do not boil miso as it can get very bitter and this destroys the living bacteria and enzymes. In Oriental medicine, miso has been used in the treatment of arthritis, colitis, diabetes and hypoglycemia; for tobacco problems; and to assist in breast feeding. It is a great afternoon drink for those who suffer from late afternoon or post-work symptoms like headache, dizziness, irritability, or general low energy."

Elson M. Haas, M.D.

✧✧✧✧✧✧✧

"With the contemporary concern over x-rays and other forms of environmental radiation, you should know that both miso and seaweed are said to act in the body to help rid it of radiation, heavy metals like lead and strontium, and other toxic substances. In Hiroshima after the bombings, one hospital which served miso every day to all its patients observed a much lower incidence of radiation sickness and death than in the general population or at other hospitals."

Elson M. Haas, M.D.

✧✧✧✧✧✧✧

"Tomatoes are not recommended for regular consumption, for they contain too much potassium and oxalic acid. It is oxalic acid which is responsible for melting down the calcium in our bones and bringing about gall and kidney stones. Taken occasionally by people with much stored animal protein, it will help to eliminate the undesirable excess."

Naboru Muramoto

✧✧✧✧✧✧✧

Tempuna

Prep Time: 20 minutes

This recipe is adapted from The New Farm Cookbook.. *It is a great substitute for tuna salad.*

8 oz. tempeh
4 scallions
½ cup sliced almonds, roasted
2 stalks celery, chopped
¼ cup chopped dill pickles
½ tsp. seasalt
dash black pepper

salad dressing:
1 cup silken tofu
¼ cup canola oil
½ tsp. seasalt

1. Steam tempeh for 15 minutes.
2. Meanwhile, chop celery, onions and pickles.
3. Roast almonds over moderate heat, stirring constantly, until fragrant.
4. Blend ingredients to make salad dressing.
5. Crumble cooled tempeh into medium-sized bowl.
6. Add remaining ingredients and salad dressing.
7. Mix well.

Serving Size and suggestions: Serve with bread for sandwiches or crackers for dipping.

Variations: To vary the flavors in this dish, simply use different flavored vinegars. Balsamic, red wine vinegar, would both be great!

༄༄༄༄༄༄༄༄༄

✿✿✿✿✿✿✿

"Any work you do for a selfless purpose, without thought of profit, is actually a form of prayer, which unifies our fragmented energy and attention and calms the mind."
　　　　　　　　　　Laurel Robertson et al.," Laurel's Kitchen"

✿✿✿✿✿✿✿

Scrumptious Soups

Cabbage Soup

Prep Time: 15 minutes
Cooking Time: 1 hour

The local Max's Operahouse Café, serves a delicious cabbage soup that my husband and I adore. This recipe is my inspired meatless version.

28 oz. canned tomatoes with juice
1 carrot, sliced
1 cup tomato juice
½ head of large green cabbage, chopped
1 large yellow onion, chopped
½ cup barley
1 cup golden raisins
2 Tbsp. dry vegetarian chicken broth
5 ¼ cups water
seasalt and pepper to taste
1 Tbsp. dried parsley
1 bay leaf
1-2 Tbsp. olive oil

1. Sauté chopped onion in olive oil in large soup pot.
2. Add tomatoes and juice; stir vegetarian chicken broth into water and add to pot.
3. Add carrot, cabbage, barley, bay leaf, parsley, salt, and pepper.
4. Bring to a boil, reduce to simmer.
5. Simmer for 30 minutes.
6. Add raisins.

7. Cook for another 30 minutes or more.
8. Serve hot.

Serving Size and suggestions: Serves 6.

Creamy Squash and Potato Soup

Prep Time: 15 minutes
Cooking Time: 40 minutes

When you are craving something warming on a cold winter night, cook up a batch of this soup. It will warm you all the way through!

  1 small kabocha or butternut squash
  1 small onion, chopped
  1 medium sweet potato or yam, orange-fleshed
  1 medium russet potato
  2 Tbsp. canola oil
  1 tsp. dried sweet basil
  4-5 cups water
  ½ cup soymilk
  sprinkle seasalt and white pepper

1. Wash, peel and chop squash and potatoes.
2. Chop onion, sauté in oil in a large soup pot.
3. Add squash to sauté.
4. Add basil, salt and pepper and sauté for 5 minutes more.
5. Add water, bring to a boil and simmer for 10 minutes.
6. Add potatoes, cook for 20-30 minutes until all vegetables are soft.
7. Remove from heat.
8. Add soymilk.
9. Blend until smooth and serve.

Serving Size and suggestions: Serves 6.

Flame Carrot Dish

Prep time: 30 minutes
Cooking time: 20 minutes

Yo'el, my son, has been telling me for a year that he will be a chef when he grows up. This summer he began truly creating his own recipes. Here is one of them. It demonstrates his love for carrots. The name is inspired by the thought of roasted carrots.

4 small-medium carrots, cubed
1 onion, chopped
¼ cup garlic oil
2 carrots, sliced
1 head broccoli, in large pieces
6 cups water
6 Tbsp. dry vegetarian chicken broth
1 clove garlic, minced
2 Tbsp. fresh Italian parsley, chopped
2 Tbsp. fresh sweet basil, chopped

1. Preheat oven to 400°. Roast the 4 chopped carrots and the onion on a baking sheet in the garlic oil for about 20 minutes. Stir regularly to avoid sticking.
2. Meanwhile, put garlic, broccoli, herbs, water and chicken broth in large soup pot, after soup begins to boil, lower heat to medium-low and simmer and cook for about 10 minutes.
3. Add roasted carrots and onions and raw sliced carrots to soup.
4. Cook for 20 minutes to blend the flavors and serve.

Serving size and suggestions: Makes about 6 servings.

Delicious Delicata Squash Barley Soup

Prep Time: 15 minutes
Cooking Time: 1 hour

This scrumptious soup makes a meal that will warm any winter night while being rich in nutritious foods.

2-3 cups delicata squash, peeled and cut in squares
6 small-medium carrots, shredded
1 cup barley
½ head green cabbage, chopped
½ daikon radish, shredded
2 stalks celery, chopped
1 tsp. Dried orange peel
handful of wakame seaweed
6-7 cups water.

1. Place water in large soup pot and bring to a boil.
2. Add barley, turn down to simmer for 20 minutes.
3. Meanwhile, prepare vegetables.
4. Add vegetables after barley cooking time is done.
5. Simmer another 20 minutes.
6. Add orange peel. Turn off heat. Serve after five minutes.

Serving Size and suggestions: Serves 6.

To make dried orange peel: Grate orange peel onto plate. Spread evenly over plate surface. Leave out to dry for a few days. Stir occasionally and spread evenly again to avoid molding. When dry, store in empty spice bottle. Lemon peel can be prepared the same way.

Variations: Use dried lemon peel instead of orange. Try different types of winter squash instead of the delicata: butternut or kabocha would both be great. Vary grains and seaweeds for a totally different soup!

Garlic Soup

Prep Time: 15 minutes
Cooking Time: 20 minutes

I had a delightful soup similar to this in a local Mexican restaurant and wanted to create a dairy-free version to warm our bellies at home.

1 spring onion or 2 leeks, chopped
8-10 small garlic cloves, minced
1 lb. russet potatoes, peeled and cubed
2 Tbsp. canola oil
4 cups water
1 tsp. seasalt
1 cup soymilk
2 cups water
2 Tbsp. dry vegetarian chicken broth
½ tsp. white pepper
herb croutons

1. Heat canola oil in large soup pot. Sauté onion or leek and garlic until soft.
2. Add dry broth to 2 cups boiling water.
3. Pour broth, remaining 2 cups of water, potatoes, salt and pepper into pot.
4. Bring to a boil, turn to simmer.
5. Simmer for 20 minutes.
6. Blend until smooth either in blender or with hand-held cuisinart.

7. Add soymilk and mix well.
8. Serve with herb croutons.

Serving Size and suggestions: Serves 3. Look for a crunchy, flavorful crouton at your local health food store. The best ones are from local bakeries.

Lentil Bean Carrot, Good for You, Yummy to Eat Soup

Prep Time: 30 minutes
Cooking Time: 30 Minutes

This dish was named by my 6 ½ year old son who couldn't get enough of it!

¾ c. TVP (textured vegetable protein)
1 tsp. cumin
1 tsp. garlic powder
1 c. lentils
1 Tbsp. soy sauce
1 carrot
1 medium white onion
2 medium tomatoes, cut in small pieces
1 tsp. curry powder
dash salt and pepper
2 ribs celery
6 Tbsp. vegetarian chicken broth, mixed with 5 c. water
½ tsp. cumin
2 Tbsp. olive oil

1. Boil one cup water and stir into TVP with cumin and garlic powder. Set aside for 10-15 minutes while water is absorbed.
2. Chop onion, carrot and celery and sauté in olive oil over medium heat until onion is translucent, about 5 minutes.

3. Rinse lentils thoroughly.
4. Add 2 cups broth to sautéed vegetables.
5. Break kombu into little pieces over vegetables and broth.
6. Add TVP, lentils, soy sauce, salt and pepper, curry, cumin, tomatoes, and 3 cups of broth.
7. Cover and simmer over medium-low heat for 30 minutes until lentils are fully cooked.
8. If you would like to make this more like a stew, open the cover to allow the steam to escape during cooking.

Serving Size and suggestions: Makes about 6 servings.

Seaweed Soup

Prep Time: 10 minutes
Cooking Time: 40 minutes

There was a Buddhist restaurant around the corner that served totally vegetarian Chinese foods using fresh ingredients and a large variety of meatless dishes that simulated meat. I loved it, as did my family, and we were all sad when it closed. In the midst of a craving for their soothing seaweed soup, I created this recipe. I find it just as soothing. I just miss being served when I'm in the need to relax and rejuvenate. This soup will do it for you too. Enjoy.

6 cups water
2" x 2" piece of kombu seaweed
2 small carrots, sliced
4 dried shiitake (black) mushrooms
1 sheet nori seaweed
½ sheet dried laver seaweed
12 oz. firm silken tofu
1 onion, in pieces (not chopped)
1-2 Tbsp. toasted sesame oil
white miso, 1 tsp. per bowl
1 scallion, chopped (optional)

1. Put sesame oil in large soup pot.
2. Sauté onion and celery in oil over med-hi heat for 2-3 minutes.
3. Add carrots and sauté for 2-3 minutes.

4. Add water and kombu, cut into small pieces.
5. Add mushrooms.
6. Cook for 20 minutes over low heat.
7. Remove the mushrooms, take off and discard the stems, slice into thin strips and return to the soup.
8. Cut tofu into small squares and add to the soup.
9. Fold nori in half, three times and cut into strips with scissors into the soup pot.
10. Cut the laver into small pieces over the soup pot.
11. Cook over low heat for 15 minutes.
12. To serve, put miso in individual bowl. Ladle a little broth into bowl and mix in miso.
13. Fill bowl with soup. Add scallions if desired.

Serving Size and suggestions: Serves 6-8. Serve with Black Soybean Sauté (page 159) and brown rice.

Variations: Use different types of seaweed. For a different effect, add 1 beaten egg at the last minute, and stir slowly into soup.

Sweet Autumn Soup

Prep Time: 10 minutes
Cooking Time: 30 minutes

This delicious soup is great to beat sugar cravings. It is naturally sweet, warm and filling.

1 yellow onion, chopped
1 ½ large butternut squash, peeled and chopped
1 medium sweet potato, peeled and chopped
1 Tbsp. canola oil
5-6 cups water
½ - 1 cup soymilk

1. Prepare onion, squash and sweet potato.
2. Sauté onion in large soup pot.
3. Add squash to onions and add a little water to lightly steam squash.
4. Stir occasionally for 10-15 minutes over low heat.
5. Add sweet potato and continue cooking on low, adding water if necessary to avoid burning or sticking. Stir to prevent sticking.
6. When vegetables are soft, after 15 minutes or so, add the rest of the water and soymilk to taste.
7. Heat until simmering again.
8. Blend a little at a time in a blender or use a cuisinart to blend soup until smooth and creamy.

Serving Size and suggestions: Serves 6. Delicious with Baked Fish with Creamy Cabbage (page 133) or Crustless Tofu Quiche (page 161).

༄༅༄༅༄༅༄༅༄༅

✧✧✧✧✧✧✧✧

"The Middle Way"
" *Shakyamuni lived many years as a wandering ascetic, going without food or water until he was reduced to skin and bone. At last, weary of these exertions, he took food and sat under a pipal tree, vowing not to move until he had found Enlightenment. All night long he was plagued with demons, but as day broke he achieved his goal and attained Nirvana. As Buddha, he went on to preach the wisdom of the middle path, between the extremes of indulgence and self-mortification."*
Lucy Lidell et al., "The Sivananda Companion to Yoga"

✧✧✧✧✧✧✧✧

Vegetable Rice Soup

Prep Time: 20 minutes
Cooking Time: 45 minutes

This is the first meal my then-to-be husband cooked for me. I was sick and needed nurturing. He made this soup for me and it definitely propelled me into wellness. I have since made some minor variations from his version.

½ head cauliflower, cut in pieces
1 carrot, sliced
4-5 leaves of greens (collard, chard, kale), shredded
1 small head broccoli, cut in pieces
½ cup brown rice
1 cup mushrooms, sliced in half
1 4"piece kombu or 1 sheet nori seaweed, crumbled
1 onion, sliced or chopped
5-6 cups water
barley miso, 1 tsp. added to each bowl at serving
Croutons or Israeli soup nuts, optional

1. Prepare vegetables as ingredient list suggests.
2. Pour water into large soup pot.
3. Add vegetables and rice to water.
4. Cover pot and bring water to boil. Turn down to simmer and cook for about half an hour. Check regularly to make sure vegetables do not get too soft.

5. When ready to serve, place 1 tsp. miso in each serving bowl. Pour a small amount of broth into bowl and stir until miso is dissolved. Ladle the rest of the soup to fill the bowl and serve.
6. Serve croutons or soup nuts in a bowl on the side.

Serving Size and suggestions: Serves 8.

Variations: Try other vegetables like parsnips, roma tomatoes, green beans, zucchini; add 5 Tbsp. dry vegetarian chicken broth instead of using miso. Experiment with spices: oregano, thyme, rosemary, basil, marjoram, seasalt and pepper.

✡✡✡✡✡✡✡

"Full of prana, a pure and moderated diet is the best possible guarantee of physical and mental health, bringing harmony and vitality to both body and mind."
    Lucy Lidell et al., "The Sivananda Companion to Yoga"

✡✡✡✡✡✡✡

Basic Beans

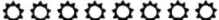

✿✿✿✿✿✿✿

"A person with a healthy way of thinking does not try to separate himself from the world of bacteria. He knows that microbes and viruses too have their purpose and are beneficial to man. They are not our enemies, they are contained in our very life - in the food we eat and in the water we drink. And they cannot harm a person in good health. It is an ancient Oriental belief that disease destroys only those who deserve it. Science's anti-microbe attitude has developed as a result of modern man's inability to make himself stronger in body and mind."
Naboru Muramoto

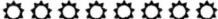

Aduki Beans with Kombu

Prep Time: 10 minutes
Cooking Time: 1 ½ hours

These beans are very easy to cook and make a delicious broth. They are excellent as a tonic for kidney health.

1 cup aduki beans
3-4 inch piece of kombu seaweed
splash soy sauce or tamari
3-4 cups water

1. Wash beans thoroughly.
2. Place all ingredients in a pot, breaking kombu into small pieces.
3. Cover and bring to a boil.
4. Lower heat to simmer for about 1 hour and 15-30 minutes.
5. Stir occasionally.
6. Beans are ready when soft.

Serving Size and suggestions: Serves 4. Delicious with Creamy Squash and Potato Soup (page 95) and cornbread.

Barbecue Baked Beans

Prep Time: soak beans overnight; next day cook beans about two hours.
Cooking Time: one hour, 20 minutes

I love this dish on a hot summer's day with the all-American picnic fixin's!

2 cups dried navy beans (5-6 cups canned)
¾ cup vegetarian bacon bits
¼ cup brown sugar
¼ cup apple cider vinegar
1 small yellow onion, chopped
1 cup barbecue sauce (your favorite)
¼ cup maple syrup
1 Tbsp. dijon mustard
½ Tbsp. salt
canola oil

1. Soak beans overnight in a large bowl with water well covering the beans. If using canned beans, skip to #3.
2. Drain the beans and add fresh water with salt. Cook for about two hours or until soft.
3. Meanwhile, sauté onion in oil. Add bacon bits, sugar, syrup and vinegar. Cook for 5 minutes.
4. Add barbecue sauce and mustard.
5. Drain beans when cooked.
6. Preheat oven to 325°.
7. Place beans in deep casserole and mix in sauce.

8. Bake covered for one hour. Add water as necessary to maintain moistness while baking.
9. Uncover and bake for twenty more minutes.

Serving Size and suggestions: Serves 8 easily. Serve with potato salad, Crustless Tofu Quiche (page 161), Cool Beet Salad (page 81) and Honey Lemonade (page 217) for a wonderful summer meal!

✺✺✺✺✺✺✺

"Cereals (or grains) are the most suitable food for man."
Naboru Muramoto

✺✺✺✺✺✺✺

Great Grains

Rice Pilaf

Prep Time: 15 minutes
Cooking Time: 40 minutes

This recipe is an adaptation of my mother's rice pilaf. It's delicious as a different grain dish when you're tired of the same old steamed brown rice.

1 cup brown rice
1 Tbsp. canola oil
1 small onion, chopped
2 stalks celery, chopped
3 Tbsp. pine nuts
2 cups water
1 Tbsp. dry vegetarian chicken broth
¼ tsp. each seasalt, pepper
1 tsp. dried parsley

1. Lightly brown rice, onion and celery in oil.
2. Sauté until onion is translucent.
3. Add broth to water and add to sauté.
4. Add spices.
5. Cover and cook for 20 minutes.
6. Add pine nuts and cook until water is absorbed, about 20 minutes.

Serving Size and suggestions: Serves 4.

Variations: Substitute bulgur or couscous for brown rice.

Couscous Pilaf

Prep Time: 10 minutes
Cooking Time: 20 minutes

  2 cups couscous
  1 large onion, chopped
  4 cups vegetable broth or water
  ½ tsp. each thyme, sage and white pepper
  1-2 Tbsp. canola or olive oil

1. Chop onion.
2. Sauté onion in oil in a large sauté pan until translucent.
3. Add couscous and sauté for two minutes.
4. Add broth or water and spices and mix well. Stir occasionally while cooking over low heat until broth is fully absorbed.

Serving Size and suggestions: Serves 6-8.

Variations: Use quinoa or millet instead of couscous.

Quinoa-Bulgur Pilaf

Prep Time: 10 minutes
Cooking Time: 20-25 minutes

Another yummy grain dish. These grains have a similar cooking time, don't try this with just any grains because you will end up with one well done and the other undercooked. Simple and quick. Enjoy!

½ cup quinoa
½ cup bulgur
2 Tbsp. dry vegetarian chicken broth
2 tsp. dried parsley
¼ cup sunflower seeds
1 onion, chopped
2 cups water
1 Tbsp. olive oil
seasalt and black pepper to taste

1. Sauté chopped onion in oil in a medium pot for 2-3 minutes.
2. Add the sunflower seeds for 2 minutes more.
3. Add water to chicken broth and mix well.
4. Add to the pot and mix well.
5. Mix in grains, parsley, seasalt and pepper.
6. Cover and bring to a boil.
7. Lower to simmer and simmer for 20-25 minutes or until water is absorbed.
8. Fluff with a fork and serve.

Serving Size and suggestions: Serves 4. Delicious with Baked Eggplant Feta (page 131) and Red Veggie Surprise (page 141).

※※※※※※※※

✿✿✿✿✿✿✿

"It is important to chew all food thoroughly. Chewing is a sacred act by which we can prevent most diseases. When we chew well, we are more careful and thoughtful with the food we are eating. Giving thoughtful consideration to each spoonful or dish is a worthwhile habit to develop. In the act of chewing we show our care and gratitude for both the food and our body."

Naboru Muramoto

✿✿✿✿✿✿✿

Simple Spanish Rice

Prep Time: 5 minutes
Cooking Time: 45 minutes

I was craving Spanish rice one night to go with my burritos and didn't know how to make it. This recipe was the result of my need for something simple and delicious.

1 cup brown rice
½ cup your favorite salsa, more to taste
2 cups water
½ lime, juiced

1. Place water, rice and salsa into a pot.
2. Bring to a boil and reduce heat to simmer.
3. Simmer until rice is completely cooked, about 45 minutes.
4. Remove from heat and add lime juice. Mix well and serve.

Serving Size and suggestions: Serves 4. Excellent with Crustless Tofu Quiche or as a side for Mexican-style Pasta Casserole.

Variations: Use lemon juice instead of lime.

Dry Lunch

Prep Time: 20 minutes
Cooking Time: 45 minutes

My husband and I came up with this excellent solution to boring bag lunches when we wanted to bring healthy food to our office for lunch. I hope you enjoy it too.

- 1/3 - ½ cup grain (brown rice, bulgur, millet…)
- 1 ½ cups water
- 2 cups cut veggies (broccoli, carrots, cauliflower, onion…)
- 1-2 tsp. miso, red, barley or white
- tamari or soy sauce to taste

1. Place dry ingredients into a casserole dish. This can be kept refrigerated for 3-4 days until ready to use.
2. Add boiling water to casserole dish and bake at 350° for 45 minutes.
3. Add tamari and miso. Mix well and serve.

Serving Size and suggestions: Serves 2.

Variations: To turn this into a soup, simply add a total of 4 cups of water.

✧✧✧✧✧✧✧

*"It is a basic need of humanity to be in touch
with the earth,
and any nation or civilization which is cut off
from it slowly
but surely loses its vigor and degenerates."*

Vinoba Bhave
spiritual successor to Mahatma Gandhi

✧✧✧✧✧✧✧

Casseroles and Other Stuff

৵৵৵৵৵৵৵৵৵৵৵৵৵৵৵

Layered Enchilada Casserole

Prep Time: 30 minutes
Cooking Time: 20-30 minutes

This casserole is a simple and cheeseless dish that takes the place beautifully of the time-consuming, meat-filled traditional enchilada. Simply delicious! This is a large casserole, so if you want to cut it in half it works just as well. You may want to make the whole thing and freeze half for a quick supper.

- 1 sm. green or yellow pepper
- 1 medium zucchini, cut in pieces
- 1 cup corn (frozen or fresh off the cob)
- 3 Tbsp. fresh parsley, chopped
- 1 medium onion, chopped
- 1 cup black olives, sliced
- ¾ cup TVP (textured vegetable protein)
- 1 cup boiling water
- 10-12 corn tortillas
- 3 Tbsp. canola oil (plus to oil pan)
- seasonings: granular garlic, chili powder, granular onion to taste

Sauce:
- 28 oz. can chunky tomato sauce
- 15 oz. can tomato sauce
- salt and pepper to taste
- 1 tsp. cumin
- 1 tsp. chili powder

1. Preheat oven to 350°.
2. Boil water and stir into TVP with the garlic, onion and chili powder to taste. Stir well. Let sit while preparing vegetables.
3. Oil 9x13 baking pan. Set aside.
4. Mix sauce ingredients together and mix well.
5. Sauté pepper, onion, TVP and parsley in oil until vegetables are soft. Add zucchini and corn and cover for 5 minutes.
6. Meanwhile, put a layer of tortillas in the oiled pan.
7. Spoon some sauce over the tortillas.
8. Add sliced olives to cooked vegetables.
9. Stir one cup of sauce into vegetables and mix well.
10. Spread vegetable mixture evenly over tortillas.
11. Cover with remaining tortillas.
12. Use remaining sauce to completely cover tortillas.
13. Bake uncovered for 20-30 minutes.

Serving Size and suggestions: Serves 8. Serve with guacamole and shredded lettuce and Simple Spanish Rice (page 121).

Variations: Use winter vegetables like broccoli and cauliflower instead of zucchini.

Green Bean and Mushroom Casserole

Prep Time: 2o minutes
Cooking Time: 30 minutes

This wholesome summer dish was inspired by my desire to have a healthy version of the old canned mushroom soup and canned green beans that were so popular in college. I replaced all the canned ingredients with fresh, added a dairy-free cream sauce and topped the whole thing with the same crunchy onions that I find at the store. This is one of the few places that I use canned items from a regular grocery supplier. Oh, well, it's okay to do occasionally.

White sauce:
2 Tbsp. whole wheat pastry flour
1 cup soymilk
2 Tbsp. butter or margarine
¼ tsp. salt
white pepper, dash
soy sauce, splash
white pepper, dash

6 oz. mushrooms, sliced
4 cups green beans, washed and in pieces
1 Tbsp. canola oil
1 medium onion, chopped
1 small can fried onions

1. Cut and stem green beans, breaking into bite-sized pieces. Steam for 5-10 minutes or until tender and still crunchy. Blanching is another good way to prepare the beans.
2. Prepare white sauce by melting the butter in a medium nonstick pan. Meanwhile heat the soy milk without scalding. Add flour to melted butter and stir constantly over medium-low heat for about 3 minutes. Add the heated soymilk slowly to the melted butter and flour (roux). Stir continuously and bring to a boil to thicken. Set aside.
3. Sauté mushrooms and onion in canola oil and add to white sauce.
4. Add a splash of soy sauce and a dash of white pepper to taste.
5. Mix green beans and white sauce together in a bowl.
6. Lightly oil a casserole and preheat the oven to 350°.
7. Pour green beans and sauce into casserole and bake for 25 minutes, uncovered.
8. Spread fried onions over the top and bake for 5 more minutes.

Serving Size and suggestions: Easily serves eight as a side dish. I like serving this with vegetarian chicken sticks and mashed or baked potatoes. Also a nice addition to the Thanksgiving Feast.

Corn Casserole

Prep Time: 20 minutes
Cooking Time: 30-35 minutes

On occasion, I do use eggs and Italian cheese. This is one of those occasions and it's well worth the wait! This casserole is a great dish for using up extra summer vegetables. It's festive and makes a wonderful pot luck favorite.

2 Tbsp. butter
1 medium onion, chopped
3 cups corn kernels (2 corn cobs)
1 cup grated zucchini
1/3 cup chopped green olives
2 medium tomatoes, chopped
1 medium green pepper, chopped
1 medium sweet red pepper, chopped
¼ cup nutritional yeast
1/3 cup cornmeal
¾ cup grated asiago cheese
3 eggs, beaten
¼ tsp. Ground turmeric
½ tsp. Dijon mustard
½ cup water
 salt and pepper to taste
½ tsp. Chili powder

1. Steam the corn on the cob. Set aside to cool.
2. Meanwhile, melt butter in a skillet until foamy.
3. Sauté onion in butter until translucent.
4. Add chopped red and green peppers and sauté together until lightly browned.
5. Cut corn off cob into a large mixing bowl.
6. Preheat oven to 350°.
7. Add beaten eggs, sautéed vegetables, chopped tomatoes, grated zucchini, nutritional yeast, cornmeal, olives, cheese, water and spices.
8. Mix thoroughly and pour into a well-oiled casserole. Bake for 30-35 minutes.

Serving Size and suggestions: Serves 6. I like to have a crisp green salad and toast with this casserole.

Baked Eggplant Feta

Prep Time: ½ hour
Cooking Time: ½ hour

My husband wanted eggplant for dinner, but couldn't say exactly what he was craving. So I rummaged around in the kitchen until I found some extra stuff that needed using up. This recipe was the delicious result! He was satisfied and so was I.

1 globe eggplant
½ cup grated asiago or soy parmesan cheese
6-8 oz. pesto
1/3 # Bulgarian feta cheese
15 oz. can Muir Glen pizza sauce
½ cup sliced black olives

1. Slice eggplant to ¼ " thickness.
2. Place on cookie sheet.
3. Spread ½ of pesto so each piece of eggplant is well-covered.
4. Broil for 10-15 minutes or until eggplant is soft and lightly browned.
5. Turn eggplant over and spread the rest of the pesto over the eggplant pieces.
6. Broil 5-8 minutes more until lightly browned on the second side.
7. Preheat oven to 350°.
8. Place half of the eggplant into a casserole dish.

9. Top the eggplant with half of the pizza sauce, half of the olives, and crumble half of the feta evenly over the top.
10. Sprinkle half of the grated cheese on top and repeat #7-9 for a second layer.
11. Cover and bake for 20 minutes. Turn off the oven and uncover for 5 minutes.

Serving Size and suggestions: Serves 4 hungry people. Garlic bread is a must!

Baked Fish with Creamy Cabbage

Prep Time: ½ hour
Cooking Time: 1 hour, 15 minutes

Normally a very rich dish with pork chops and cream, I have lightened this dish up by using soymilk and fresh fish instead. Delicious! You can also make this dish without the fish for a delicious vegetarian meal.

 1 large head green cabbage, shredded
 4 pieces, 2-3" thick fresh tuna or swordfish
 ½ cup chopped onions
 ½ cup cooking Sherry wine
 1 cup soymilk
 2 tsp. dry bread crumbs
 3 Tbsp. butter or margarine
 ½ tsp. minced garlic
 4 Tsp. grated parmesan cheese
 3 Tbsp. canola or olive oil
 1 bay leaf
 ½ tsp. each seasalt and black pepper

1. Steam shredded cabbage in large steamer until it is wilted.
2. Melt 2 Tbsp. of butter over medium heat in a large skillet.
3. Cook onions and garlic for 3-4 minutes, stirring constantly.

4. Stir cabbage into skillet. Add seasalt and pepper and cook for 5 minutes, stirring frequently.
5. Transfer vegetables to a bowl, and set aside.
6. In the same skillet, melt 1 Tbsp. butter and add oil.
7. Lightly brown the fish in the skillet. Set aside.
8. Pour off excess fats, add wine and boil rapidly, until reduced to ¼ cup.
9. Mix wine into cabbage.
10. Spread 1/2 of cabbage in deep casserole dish. Lay browned fish on top of cabbage and layer the rest of the cabbage over fish.
11. Scald soymilk (look for tiny bubbles at edge) in small pan and pour over fish and cabbage, adding bay leaf to top.
12. Place casserole on baking sheet, cover with lid and bake at 350° for 1 hour.
13. Mix parmesan cheese and bread crumbs. Remove lid sprinkle mixture on top and bake for 15 minutes.

Serving Size and suggestions: Serves 4. Bulgur Pilaf (page 117) is an excellent side dish.

Stuffed Steamed Greens

Prep Time: 1 hour
Cooking Time: 30 minutes

I returned from a trip to New York in early June, and found an enormous quantity of the biggest greens I have ever grown in my garden. I almost didn't recognize what they were! This tantalizing recipe created itself during my yoga class.

   1 small zucchini
   1 small peter pan squash
   1 small yellow summer squash
   1 medium carrot
   8 large leaves chard or collard greens
   1 Tbsp. soy sauce
   1 Tbsp. dry vegetarian chicken broth
   1 recipe quinoa-bulgur pilaf (page 119) or
rice pilaf (page 117)

1. Start rice pilaf, stopping at step 5 when the rice is cooking.
2. While the rice is cooking, wash the greens.
3. Place the greens in layers in a steamer basket and steam for 5 minutes (after water begins to boil in steamer).
4. Meanwhile cut carrots and squashes into small cubes.
5. Boil 2 cups of water and blanche the vegetables in the water for 5 minutes.

6. Drain veggies and mix into pilaf when rice is fully cooked. Add soy sauce and mix well.
7. Allow greens and pilaf to cool.
8. Carefully remove the greens from the basket and place with spine-side down onto cutting board, open flat.
9. Spread about ½ cup of pilaf-veggie mix onto center of leaf along the spine.
10. Fold over the left and right edges of the leaf into the center.
11. Fold up the stem end into the center, and roll over once more to complete folding.
12. Place folded side down into large casserole and repeat with the rest of the leaves. You may have some pilaf-veggie mix left over.
13. Mix dry chicken broth into 1 cup water and stir well.
14. Pour broth into edges of casserole around the stuffed leaves.
15. Cover and bake at 350° for 30 minutes.

Serving Size and suggestions: Serves 6-8 depending on their appetites. Excellent served with the Israeli Cut Salad (page 85) and fresh bread.

Stuffed Squash

Prep Time: 45 minutes
Cooking Time: 20-30 minutes

My garden had a particularly abundant crop of winter squash and greens one year, so I created this dish to use some of the extras. I use my husband's homemade soysage in this dish, but the store-bought varieties are great too!

   2 medium butternut squash
   1 cup bulgur
   1 bunch greens (spinach, collards, kale…)
   1 cup vegetarian sausage
   1 large onion
   2 -3 Tbsp. olive oil
   1 large onion, chopped
   dried parsley, to taste
   ¼ cup nutritional yeast
   1 large tomato, chopped
   2 cups water

1. Preheat oven to 350°
2. Cut squash in half and steam until soft when pierced with a fork.
3. Meanwhile, cook bulgur in 2 cups water until done.
4. Cool steamed squash and scoop out squash, leaving ½" around the edges.
5. Chop onion and tomato, wash and chop greens and crumble sausage.

6. Sauté onion and sausage in oil for 2 minutes over medium heat.
7. Add greens and sauté until greens are wilted, adding oil if needed.
8. Stir cooked squash into sausage mix, add tomatoes, parsley and nutritional yeast.
9. Remove from heat and mix with bulgur.
10. Stuff mixture into squash shells and bake for 20-30 minutes or until lightly browned on top.

Serving Size and suggestions: Makes four large servings when shells are cut in half after baking. Serve with Aduki Beans with Kombu (page 112) and a green salad.

Roasted Winter Vegetables

Prep Time: 15 minutes
Cooking Time: 45 minutes

This is a very simple dish and has a gourmet quality to it.

- 1 large onion, sliced
- 1 head cauliflower, in pieces
- 1 parsnip, cubed
- 2 large stalks broccoli, in pieces
- 4 medium red or Yellow Finn potatoes, cubed
- 2 carrots, cubed
- ½ cup sliced pimento-stuffed green olives
- ½ cup sliced kalamata olives
- dash seasalt and pepper
- 2-3 garlic cloves
- olive oil
- 1-2 Tbsp. balsamic vinegar

1. Preheat oven to 400°.
2. Generously coat baking sheet with olive oil. Add minced garlic and spread evenly.
3. Place prepared vegetables on baking sheet and stir until lightly coated with oil.
4. Sprinkle with salt and pepper.
5. Bake for about 35 minutes, until vegetables are completely cooked and shrunken considerably. Stir regularly so that vegetables do not stick to baking sheet.

6. Add olives, stir well and bake for 10 minutes.
7. Remove from oven and sprinkle with balsamic vinegar. Mix well and serve.

Garlic Oil :To make pour a generous amount of olive oil into an empty jar. Peel three garlic cloves and cut in half. Drop garlic into olive oil and refrigerate. In about one week the oil will become infused with garlic flavor. The longer it is left in the refrigerator, the stronger the garlic becomes.

Serving Size and suggestions: Serves 6. Excellent with Bulgur Pilaf (page 117) or Rice Pilaf (page 117) and Baked Tofu (page 163). See Pita with Roasted Vegetables (page 61).

Variations: Use seasonal vegetables for a year-round meal (mushrooms, eggplant, green beans, corn, tomatoes, green peppers). Choose your favorite combinations and have fun!

Red Veggie Surprise

Prep Time: 10 minutes
Cooking Time: 15 minutes

This is a dish that was born of that time between the last of the winter vegetables and the beginning of spring vegetables.

1 large parsnip, cut in sticks
1 large beet, cut in sticks
1 large carrot, cut in sticks
1 bunch asparagus, cut in pieces
1 small onion, chopped
1 Tbsp. sesame seeds
1 ½ cups boiling water
2 Tbsp. canola oil
1 ½ Tbsp. sliced almonds
¼ cup dry vegetarian chicken broth

1. Sauté onion in oil for 2 minutes.
2. Add parsnip, beet and carrot for 2 minutes.
3. Add boiling water mixed with chicken broth.
4. Bring to a boil.
5. Simmer for 10 minutes.
6. Meanwhile, roast seeds and almonds in an iron skillet, stirring constantly, for 2-3 minutes or until fragrant and lightly browned.
7. Add asparagus to veggies.
8. Simmer for 5-10 minutes.

9. Sprinkle seeds and nuts on individual servings.

Serving Size and suggestions: Serves 6. Serve with Couscous Pilaf (page 118) or Quinoa-Bulgur Pilaf (page 119) and Baked Tofu (page 163).

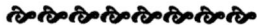

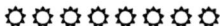

"We should consider the possibility that nature provided us with a system which appreciates simplicity and not mixing our foods. Another possibility is that foods which grow together may be eaten together."
                                                                Elson M. Haas, M.D.

✧✧✧✧✧✧✧

"You can gloomily experience every breath or change in terms of what you're losing, focusing on what you will no longer have. Or you can be open and joyful, welcoming each breath and each change in your life by looking toward the new experience and growth it will bring. When you dwell on the melancholy, you are prone to injury of the Metal element and in turn to colds, lung ailments, and digestive problems."
Elson M. Haas, M.D.

✧✧✧✧✧✧✧

Pleasing Pastas

Amy's Anything Goes Garden Pasta

Prep Time: 30 minutes
Cooking Time: 15 minutes

It seems that every good cookbook has a version of Pasta Primavera. I think it comes from the natural abundance of keeping fresh veggies around the house. Here's my version. Hope you like it!

1 medium carrot, bite-sized pieces
1 medium green zucchini, bite-sized pieces
2 roma tomatoes, chopped
1 cup green beans, bite-sized pieces
3 leaves collard greens
1 medium yellow squash, bite-sized pieces
1 onion, sliced
12 oz. fusilli pasta
3 Tbsp. olive oil
3 Tbsp. butter
1 Tbsp. lemon basil
2 Tbsp. Italian parsley
1 Tbsp. savory
2 cloves garlic, minced

1. Boil 6 cups of water in a 4 quart pot.
2. Cut vegetables. Blanche carrots, green beans, and squashes in boiling water for 5 minutes.

3. Add chopped greens for last minute of blanching.
4. Scoop vegetables out and set water aside for cooking the pasta.
5. Melt butter with olive oil in a large non-stick skillet.
6. Meanwhile, boil the reserved water and prepare pasta according to package directions.
7. Sauté the onion and garlic in the oil and butter for 3 minutes over medium-high.
8. Add the herbs and sauté for 5 minutes over medium-low.
9. Add the chopped tomatoes and sauté for 2 minutes or until the tomatoes are warmed through.
10. Serve over cooked and drained pasta with grated parmesan or asiago cheese.

Serving Size and suggestions: Serves 4.

Variations: As the name says, anything goes. So try whatever vegetable or herb combinations that sound yummy to you!

Eggplant Parmesan Lasagna

Prep Time: 30 minutes
Cooking Time: 60 minutes

Two of my favorite dishes are eggplant parmesan and lasagna. I thought it would be fun to have them both at once without eating two main dishes! Here's to having your eggplant and lasagna too!

1 eggplant, sliced thinly
12 oz. soy mozzarella, shredded
1/8 cup garlic oil
4 cups mushroom & onion marinara sauce (page 67), or your favorite store-bought sauce
½ cup soy parmesan or asiago cheese
12 oz. lasagna noodles

Tofu-Ricotta Cheese:
12.5 oz package silken tofu
2 tsp. garlic powder

1. Slice eggplant. Place on a large baking sheet and drizzle garlic oil over eggplant until well covered.
2. Broil eggplant until soft and lightly browned, but not burned, about 10 minutes.
3. Remove from oven and set aside. Preheat oven to 375°.
4. Blend tofu with garlic powder until almost smooth.

5. Spread a layer of marinara sauce, approximately 1 ½ cups, on the bottom of the pan.
6. Place a layer of the lasagna noodles, uncooked, over the sauce.
7. Put a layer of the eggplant on the lasagna.
8. Spoon a tablespoon of tofu-ricotta cheese on top of eggplant in 5 or 6 places.
9. Cover the eggplant with a layer of half of the mozzarella and half of the asiago cheeses.
10. Repeat layering, starting with the sauce again, and ending with the cheeses on top.
11. Bake the lasagna, covered, for 40 minutes.
12. Remove cover and bake for another 5-10 minutes or until cheese is lightly browned.

Serving Size and suggestions: Serve hot with garlic bread and a green salad.

Variations:
Spinach Lasagna: Steam 1 bunch well-washed spinach, without stems, until wilted and use in place of eggplant.

Sausage: Sauté 1 cup of vegetarian sausage in 1-2 Tbsp. olive oil and add to sauce or sprinkle on eggplant or spinach.

Mexican-style Pasta Casserole

Prep Time: 30 minutes
Cooking Time: 25 minutes

This is a dish that I find wonderfully warming on a cold winter night. Full of proteins and other nutrients, I love treating my tongue and my health at the same time.

1 bunch spinach, well cleaned and chopped
1 large onion, chopped
1 cup vegetarian sausage or TVP (textured vegetable protein)
1 ½ cups salsa, your favorite
1 cup corn kernels
¾ cup soy mozzarella, shredded
¾ cup soy cheddar. shredded
15 oz. tomato sauce
8 oz. bow pasta or macaroni
¼ cup sliced green olives
¼ cup sliced black olives
1 tsp. seasalt
½ tsp. oregano
2 Tbsp. canola oil

1. If using TVP, soak in ¾ cup boiling water with ¼ tsp. garlic powder. Set aside.
2. Preheat oven to 350°.
3. Prepare spinach and onion.

4. In large skillet, brown crumbled sausage or reconstituted TVP and onion in oil.
5. Add spinach and stir gently until thoroughly wilted.
6. Add salsa, tomato sauce, seasalt and oregano. Stir well and bring to a light boil.
7. Reduce to simmer and stir for a minute or two. Remove from heat.
8. Cook pasta in boiling water until done. Drain and mix into sauce.
9. Add corn kernels, sliced olives, and ¼ cup of each cheese and mix well.
10. Pour mixture into a 9" x 13" casserole. Bake for 25 minutes.
11. Top with remaining cheese. Bake for five minutes or until cheese is melted.

Serving Size and suggestions: Serves 6. Serve with shredded lettuce, tofu sour cream and guacamole. Provide extra salsa for those who like it hot!

Multi-color Pasta

Prep Time: 20 minutes
Cooking Time: 30 minutes

This is a colorful dish that deserves to be displayed at potlucks or special occasions. It is simple and delicious.

28 oz. canned peeled tomatoes
6 oz. tomato paste, Italian style
½ cup water (or more if needed)
½ cup frozen peas
½ cup frozen or fresh corn
15 oz. can kidney beans
1 medium onion, chopped
1 large garlic clove, minced
½ cup black olives, sliced
1 Tbsp. olive oil
salt and pepper to taste
1-12 oz. pasta (small shapes)

1. Chop onion and mince garlic.
2. Sauté onion and garlic in olive oil over medium heat in large sauté pan until translucent.
3. Add canned tomatoes to the sauté. Cut tomatoes into pieces while they are warming.
4. Stir tomato paste and extra water into sauté. Mix well over medium-high heat.
5. Add beans, corn, peas, olives to sauté and sprinkle with salt and pepper to taste.

6. When the sauce begins to bubble, turn to simmer and cover.
7. Cook the sauce for about 30 minutes on simmer.
8. Meanwhile, boil pasta water, add pasta and cook according to directions until done.
9. Mix cooked pasta and sauce together thoroughly and serve.

Serving Size and suggestions: Serves 6. Top with grated soy parmesan or asiago cheese.

Variations: Blanche a cup of broccoli pieces and a cup of cauliflower pieces in water to replace the peas and corn.

Spinach-Mushroom Pesto over Vermicelli

Prep Time: 20 minutes

One evening a friend dropped by to visit so I invited her to stay for dinner. I searched around to see what I could make for her to enjoy. I found leftover pesto, mushrooms that desperately needed using and a bunch of fresh spinach. So I whipped up this sauce and tried it over vermicelli noodles. She loved it! Whew!

2 spring onions, chopped
1 Tbsp. olive oil
1 bunch spinach, washed & stemmed
2 cups sliced mushrooms
1 Tbsp. pesto
12 oz. vermicelli
grated parmesan

1. Sauté spring onion and mushrooms in olive oil.
2. After 2 minutes, add pesto and mix well.
3. After 2 more minutes flatten mushrooms onto bottom of pan and top with spinach.
4. Cover pan with lid to wilt spinach.
5. Meanwhile, boil water to cook vermicelli.
6. When spinach is wilted, stir together thoroughly.
7. Mix vermicelli and sauce well and serve with grated parmesan.

Serving Size and suggestions: Serves 4. Tasty with Green Bean Salad (page 83). Follow-up with Carob Brownies with Pudding Top (page 193) for a treat.

ช่วงช่วงช่วงช่วงช่วง

✧✧✧✧✧✧✧

"By eating properly we strengthen ourselves, body and mind, so that in the event of disease we do not have to panic and put ourselves at the mercy of the first curative technique that is presented to us."
                                                                    Naboru Muramoto

✧✧✧✧✧✧✧

Tantalizing Tofu, Tempeh and TVP

Spinach Soufflé

Prep Time: half an hour
Cooking Time: 45 minutes

When I was a girl, my Mom often served a frozen spinach soufflé that I just loved. I have fond memories of it still and decided to recreate it without using eggs and still have the tantalizing crusty top with a creamy inside. It worked and here it is for you to enjoy!

3 Tbsp. butter or margarine
1 small onion, chopped
2 bunches spinach, thoroughly washed
1 package (12.5 oz) silken tofu
1 Tbsp. whole wheat pastry flour
1 Tbsp. canola oil
2 Tbsp. nutritional yeast flakes
½ cup soymilk
seasalt and pepper to taste

1. Preheat oven to 375°.
2. Wash spinach thoroughly, removing the stems.
3. Chop onion and sauté in 2 Tbsp. butter in a large skillet over medium heat stirring constantly.
4. Add spinach gradually, until you can cover the skillet.
5. Stir occasionally until spinach is wilted.
6. Blend onion and spinach with tofu with cuisinart, blender or food processor until smooth.
7. Add nutritional yeast and mix well.

8. Melt 1 Tbsp. butter in same skillet on low, add flour and stir well being very careful not to burn. When well mixed, add soymilk, salt and pepper to taste.
9. Simmer until thick, stirring regularly.
10. Pour thickened sauce into spinach blend and mix well.
11. Pour into oiled 8" square casserole. Bake uncovered for 45 minutes or until lightly browned on top.

Serving Size and suggestions: Serves 6 as a side dish with Cool Beet Salad (page 81) and Creamy Squash and Potato Soup (page 95).

Variations: For a cheesier flavor, add more nutritional yeast.

Black Soy Bean Sauté

Prep Time: 30 minutes
Cooking Time: 18 minutes

I took a class in Macrobiotic cooking and was introduced to a wonderful bean I had never had before: the black soy bean. I couldn't find it in my local store until recently when I found a can of organic black soy beans by Eden foods. I was delighted! This is the first recipe I created from my joy at finding these delectable beans.

- 1 tsp. canola oil
- 1 tsp. grated ginger
- 1 tsp. Chinese sesame oil
- 1 ½ tsp. tamari
- 1 medium clove garlic, minced
- 2 small stalks broccoli, about 2 cups in bite-sized pieces
- 1 cup corn, fresh off the cob
- 1 cup cherry 100 tomatoes
- 13 oz. firm tofu, drained and cut in cubes
- 1 - 15 oz. can black soy beans

1. Place tofu on a plate and set the plate at an angle to let the water drain off. Leave for half an hour and then cut into cubes.
2. Drain the liquid from the beans into a bowl and reserve for later.

3. Cut the corn off the cob into a bowl and measure out one cup.
4. Sauté the garlic and ginger in the sesame and canola oils in a large sauté pan over medium-high heat for one minute.
5. Add the tofu cubes and tamari for two minutes stirring continuously.
6. Add the broccoli, half of the reserved bean liquid and the beans.
7. Continue cooking on medium-high for 5 minutes.
8. Add the corn and the rest of the bean liquid and the tomatoes and cook for another ten minutes until broccoli is a deep green and everything is well heated.

Serving Size and suggestions: Serves 4. Excellent with brown rice.

Variations: Try different vegetables during different seasons. A hint: don't get carried away adding veggies, part of the joy of this dish is its simplicity.

Crustless Tofu Quiche

Prep Time: 20 minutes
Cooking Time: 40 minutes

Originally, I cooked this recipe with a homemade crust as an alternative to the high in fat and caloric meat, egg and cheese quiches. I recreated this recipe one night when I was in a hurry and had a craving for quiche. Since then I have found that others also prefer this quiche crustless. It makes a great potluck dish. Full of protein without the meat. I prefer using soy cheese when I can find one that tastes good. If you are allergic to dairy, check to be sure there is no rennet in the soy cheeses.

19-20 oz. firm tofu
1 small onion, chopped
1 small carrot, grated
1 bunch spinach
¼ - ½ lb. mushrooms (shiitake, crimini, white, your favorite)
¾ cup cheddar-style soy cheese
¼ tsp. each dried sweet basil, marjoram, sage
dash of seasalt and pepper
2 Tbsp. plus olive oil

1. Preheat oven to 400°.
2. Wash, chop and grate vegetables.
3. Grate soy cheese and set aside.

4. Sauté vegetables in 2 Tbsp. olive oil, starting with onion and mushrooms, add carrots after 2 minutes and sauté for 1 minute more.
5. Add spinach and cover with lid for 1-2 minutes or until spinach is wilted.
6. Set vegetables aside.
7. Drain tofu. Blend tofu until smooth and creamy, if too dry add a splash of soymilk or water.
8. Mix tofu, vegetables, cheese and spices in a large bowl until well mixed.
9. Lightly oil a medium-sized casserole (8x8 is good).
10. Pour quiche batter into casserole and spread until evenly distributed.
11. Bake for 40 minutes or until lightly browned and firm to the touch.

Serving Size and suggestions: Serves 6.

Variations: Replace carrots, spinach and mushrooms with ½ cup corn, 1 bunch shredded chard, 1 cubed zucchini, 1 cup cherry tomatoes sliced in half. Replace cheddar with asiago or parmesan cheese. Leave out sage. The rest is basically the same.

Baked Tofu

Prep Time: 10 minutes
Cooking Time: 45 minutes

This is a tasty dish for anytime. We take it when we travel as a great lunch or snack, for car, plane or backpacking trips. It's also exquisite served fresh and hot with grain and vegetables.

19 oz. firm tofu
1 tsp. each (more or less to taste) granulated garlic, marjoram, savory, dill, thyme
½ cup teriyaki sauce (page 173)
½ cup olive oil

1. Drain and slice tofu into thin pieces.
2. Place in a 9" x 13" baking dish.
3. Pour olive oil and teriyaki sauce over tofu until all pieces are wet.
4. Sprinkle spices lightly over tofu.
5. Bake at 350° for 40 minutes.
6. Broil until tops are brown, approximately 2 minutes.

Serving Size and suggestions: Serves 4. Great with Colorful Coleslaw (page 79) or Roasted Vegetables (page 139) and Bulgur Pilaf (page 117).

Variations: Experiment with different spices.

Barbeque Tempeh

Prep Time: overnight
Cooking Time: 15-20 minutes

Once again, I find a great food at the store and then I cannot find it again. So, I create my own version and here it is.

8 oz. tempeh
canola oil
BQ sauce (your favorite)

1. Slice tempeh into thinner pieces about ½ the thickness and 2 inches across by 3 inches long. This is an approximation, do the best you can without crumbling the tempeh.
2. Lightly grease a casserole dish with the canola oil. Don't use a lot, the sauce also keeps it from sticking.
3. Place tempeh pieces in the casserole dish.
4. Slather generously on both sides with BQ sauce.
5. Marinate overnight in the refrigerator.
6. Bake at 375° for 10 minutes on each side, or brown in a nonstick pan on the stovetop over medium heat.

Serving Size and suggestions: Makes about 8 pieces. Serve with your favorite side dishes.

Variations: Use different types of sauces: teriyaki, salad dressing marinades, sweet and sour, etc.

Early Summer Vegetables with Tempeh

Prep Time: 15 minutes
Cooking Time: 15 minutes

I got in the mood for some Chinese-style vegetables from my early summer garden. Since I also needed some protein, I threw in some tempeh. If you don't have fresh herbs, dried will work fine.

4 oz. tempeh, cut in squares
1 large carrot, sliced
1 medium yellow summer squash, sliced
2 c. purple or green bush beans in 1 ½" pieces
1 medium onion, sliced
1 Tbsp. Chinese sesame oil
2-3 Tbsp. canola oil
1 Tbsp. soy sauce
½ Tbsp. curly parsley, chopped coarsely
½ Tbsp. savory, chopped coarsely

1. Pour sesame oil and 1 Tbsp. canola oil in non-stick pan.
2. Add sliced onions and tempeh squares to pan.
3. Over medium heat, sauté for about 2-3 minutes, and occasionally turn tempeh to brown both sides.
4. Add beans, squash and carrots to onions and tempeh. Turn heat to medium-high.
5. Stir well and sprinkle soy sauce over veggies.

6. Add savory and parsley, mix well making sure nothing is sticking to pan.
7. Add 1-2 Tbsp. canola oil if necessary to keep vegetables from sticking.
8. Sauté for 5-10 minutes until beans are a bright green.

Serving Size and suggestions: Serves 4 as a main dish with steamed brown rice.

❧❧❧❧❧❧❧❧

✪✪✪✪✪✪✪

"Summer is usually hot and we are more active. We need a diet which keeps us cool and light-isn't it fortunate that nature provides us with such luscious fruits and vegetables to eat at this time? The gardens and orchards are full. A diet of primarily raw fruits and vegetables, organically grown (without pesticides and other chemicals), is ideal. This will help you feel lighter, aid in weight loss and keep your energy strong."

Elson M. Haas, M.D.

✪✪✪✪✪✪✪

Green Bean Sauté with Tempeh and Shiitakes

Prep Time: 10 minutes
Cooking Time: 10 minutes

I had an abundance of green beans from my garden and was craving shiitake mushrooms, so I thought I'd add a source of protein and call it a meal!

- 8 oz. tempeh, cut in squares
- 3 c. green beans in 1" pieces
- 10 medium shiitake mushrooms
- 2 large garlic cloves, minced
- 1 Tbsp. canola oil
- 1 Tbsp. Chinese sesame oil
- 1 Tbsp. tamari
- 2 Tbsp. slivered almonds

1. Sauté garlic with oils in a large non-stick pan over low heat for one minute.
2. Raise heat to medium-high and add green beans, mushrooms, tempeh and tamari.
3. Stir fry for 7 minutes.
4. Add almonds at the end of cooking time to heat through. Serve.

Serving Size and suggestions: Serves 6 with Sliced Tomatoes in Lemon-Basil Miso Dressing (page 87) and Couscous Pilaf (page 118).

Tempelafel Patties

Prep Time: 45 minutes
Cooking Time: 20 minutes

I love the falafel I get when visiting Israel with my husband. I thought it would be fun to add a little more protein to this delicious meal and here is what I came up with.

15 oz. can garbanzo beans
1 small yellow onion, finely chopped
1/3 cup bread crumbs
1 egg, lightly beaten
½ cup dry short grain brown rice, cooked in 1 cup water
4 oz. tempeh
½ tsp. dry basil
½ tsp. ground cumin
2 large garlic cloves, minced
canola oil

1. Preheat oven to 375°.
2. Mix all ingredients in a food processor or blender until smooth.
3. Generously oil a large baking sheet.
4. Spoon mixture onto baking sheet in 2" patties.
5. Bake in preheated oven for 10 minutes on each side.

Serving Size and suggestions: Makes about 12 patties. Serve with whole wheat pitas, sliced tomatoes, shredded lettuce and tahina.

Sesame Tempeh

Prep Time: 10 minutes
Cooking Time: 10 minutes

I had some leftover raw tempeh in the frig and didn't know what to do with it before it went bad. So while I was cooking dinner one night, I threw it into a pan and created this sensational dish.

 8 oz. tempeh
1-2 tsp. soy sauce
½ Tbsp. Chinese sesame oil

1. Cut tempeh down the middle while holding it on the side to create 2 pieces the same size only thinner.
2. Cut these two pieces into bite-size squares making 20-25 pieces.
3. In a non-stick sauté pan over medium heat, warm ¾ Tbsp. sesame oil.
4. Put half of the tempeh squares in the pan, making sure to spread the oil with the pieces to cover the bottom of the pan.
5. Sprinkle 1 tsp. soy sauce into the sauté pan, allowing some to be directly in the pan and some on the tempeh.
6. Cook tempeh 3-5 minutes on each side until golden brown.
7. Remove from pan and repeat with the second half of the tempeh.
8. Serve hot.

Serving Size and suggestions: Makes 20-25 squares. Serve as an appetizer before a Middle-Eastern meal of Tempelafel Patties (page 168), and Israeli Cut Salad (page 85).

Variations: Also delicious as a replacement for the TVP in the Sweet and Sour TVP Strips (page 171).

☙☙☙☙☙☙☙☙

Sweet and Sour TVP Strips

Prep Time: 35 minutes
Cooking Time: 20 minutes

A delicious recipe created by my husband, Ofer. If you enjoy Chinese sweet and sour but don't want to eat meat, try this one!

2 cups TVP (textured vegetable protein) strips
20 oz. pineapple chunks, use juice from this can for part of 3 cups of juice
1 red bell pepper, cut in pieces
1 medium onion, cut in pieces
1 Tbsp. sesame seeds
3 Tbsp. honey
3 Tbsp. soy sauce
3 cups pineapple juice
3 Tbsp. rice vinegar
3 Tbsp. catsup
¼ - ½ tsp. ginger powder

1. Bring to a boil the pineapple juice, vinegar, honey, catsup, soy sauce, ginger powder and onion.
2. Add the TVP strips and remove from the heat. Let TVP stand to marinate for at least a half hour.
3. Oil baking sheet with sesame oil.
4. Remove TVP from sauce and place on oiled baking sheet.
5. Broil TVP for ten minutes, stirring occasionally and then add the sesame seeds and continue to broil.

6. Meanwhile cook remaining sauce with bell pepper and pineapple chunks until soft and hot.
7. Remove bell peppers and pineapple chunks from sauce and add to baking sheet under broiler for five more minutes.
8. Broil everything until TVP is browned and crusty. Keep a close eye that you do not burn the TVP.

Serving Size and suggestions: Serves 4. Serve over brown rice with extra sauce on the side.

Variations: You can add different vegetables to this dish to make it a more lively meal. Broccoli, cauliflower, and zucchini would be great additions. Replace the TVP with the Sesame Tempeh (page 169) for a wonderful and different dish.

Teriyaki TVP and Vegetables

Prep Time: 1 hour
Cooking Time: 20 minutes

Here's a great meatless teriyaki dish that will satisfy any teriyaki lover!

- 1 ½ cup TVP (textured vegetable protein) strips
- 1 carrot, cut in thin sticks
- 1 yellow onion, sliced
- 8 oz. mung bean sprouts
- 1/3 lb. shiitake mushrooms, sliced
- 1-2 Tbsp. canola oil

Teriyaki sauce:
- ½ cup soy sauce or tamari
- 2 Tbsp. honey
- 1/3 cup mirin or sherry
- 2 medium garlic cloves, minced
- 1 Tbsp. ginger root, grated
- ¾ cup water

1. Warm sauce ingredients over medium-low heat to melt honey. Add TVP strips, stir until well-coated, remove from heat and marinate for one hour.
2. Strain TVP strips, keeping sauce aside.
3. Broil TVP on a baking sheet, watch closely and stir regularly to avoid burning. Broil for about 10 minutes.
4. Warm a wok, add oil, and stir fry onion slightly.

5. Add carrots and mushrooms. Stir fry for 5-7 minutes.
6. Add bean sprouts with ¼ cup teriyaki sauce.
7. Add broiled TVP strips and serve.

Serving Size and suggestions: Serves 4. Delicious served over brown rice with extra teriyaki on the side.

Variations: Feel free to add more of your favorite vegetables! Simply cut them into bite-sized pieces and add during the stir fry portion of the cooking.

TVP Chili

Prep Time: 10 minutes
Cooking Time: 30 - 40 minutes

For those who want the health benefits of vegetarianism and the lovely flavors of old-fashioned chili, try this one on for size! Feel free to experiment with all kinds of fresh beans instead of canned. Just be sure they are well-cooked first.

1 - 15oz. can pinto beans
1 - 15oz. can kidney beans
1 cup TVP (textured vegetable protein)
7/8 cup boiling water
½ tsp. garlic powder
1 tsp. cumin
2 tsp. seasalt
2 Tbsp. chili powder
15oz. tomato sauce
1 onion, chopped
1 clove garlic, minced
2 Tbsp. canola or olive oil
black pepper to taste
 1 cup water mixed with 2 Tbsp. dry vegetarian chicken broth
½ cup water

1. Put TVP in a small bowl with boiling water and stir well.

2. Add garlic powder, ½ tsp. chili powder, and 1 tsp. seasalt.
3. Stir well and soak for 10 minutes.
4. Sauté onion and garlic in oil in a medium-sized soup pot.
5. Add TVP and brown over medium heat for 2-3 minutes, stirring constantly so TVP doesn't stick to bottom of pot.
6. Add tomato sauce, broth, ½ cup water, 1 tsp. cumin, 1 tsp. seasalt, 1 Tbsp. chili powder (for spicy add more), and black pepper to taste.
7. Bring to a boil.
8. Lower to simmer and add beans with liquid.
9. Simmer for 20 - 30 minutes and serve.

Serving Size and suggestions: Serves 6.

✿✿✿✿✿✿✿

"Perhaps, though, the real point is not so much to find the holy places as to make them. Do we not hallow places by our very commitment to them? When we turn our home into a place that nourishes and heals and contents, we are meeting directly the hungers that a consumer society exacerbates but never satisfies."

Laurel Robertson et al., " Laurel's Kitchen"

✿✿✿✿✿✿✿

A Thanksgiving Feast

🙦🙦🙦🙦🙦🙦🙦🙦🙦🙦🙦🙦🙦🙦

I love Thanksgiving and all the fixings that go with it. As a vegetarian, I found that I could still enjoy this holiday meal without meat. I thought you might enjoy this menu as another possibility for any holiday with or without the generic turkey. By the way, vegetarian-style turkeys are now available through health food stores, so if you need to have a turkey, try this option.

Broccoli in Cheesy Sauce

Prep Time: 25 minutes
Cooking Time: 30 minutes

This is another one of those recipes that was inspired by frozen favorites from my childhood. I use soy cheese instead of regular cheese. If you are allergic to dairy, make sure the soy cheese doesn't have additives taken from dairy (casein, rennet). I hope you enjoy this delightful recipe too!

2 cups broccoli, cut in pieces
8 oz. cheddar-style soy cheese
1/3 cup nutritional yeast
2 Tbsp. butter
1 cup soymilk
2 Tbsp. whole wheat pastry flour

1. Lightly steam broccoli for about 12 minutes.
2. Preheat oven to 350°.

3. Meanwhile, melt butter over medium-low heat.
4. Add flour to melted butter and stir until well mixed forming a roux.
5. Add soymilk to roux and stir well.
6. When heated through, add yeast and stir until completely blended.
7. Add crumbled cheese.
8. Stir until mixture has thickened and cheese is melted.
9. Place steamed broccoli into casserole.
10. Pour cheese sauce over broccoli.
11. Cover and bake for 30 minutes. Remove cover and broil for 5 minutes.

Serving Size and suggestions: Serves 4.

Variations: Use cauliflower instead of broccoli, or use half of each.

Stuffing

Prep Time: 30 minutes
Cooking Time: 30 minutes

Once again I am faced with a holiday meal that is filled with foods that are less than healthy, but are considered traditional. So I have put together a delicious, meatless stuffing to be eaten without a bird.

1 ½ cups vegetarian chicken broth
½ loaf whole wheat bread, crumbled
2 ribs celery
1 small onion
4 oz. white mushrooms
¼ cup pine nuts
1 tsp. sage
1 tsp. marjoram
½ tsp. thyme
½ tsp. salt
½ tsp. pepper
1 Tbsp. olive oil

1. Chop celery, onion and mushrooms.
2. Sauté vegetables in olive oil over medium-heat in a skillet until onions are translucent and mushrooms are lightly browned.
3. Meanwhile, crumble the bread into a large bowl.
4. Mix sautéed vegetables into bread crumbs.
5. Add pine nuts and spices.

6. Mix well.
7. Add broth and mix thoroughly.
8. Bake at 350° for 30 minutes.

Serving Size and suggestions: Serves 6.
Variations: Vary mushrooms and nuts to create unusual dishes.

Maple Cranberries

Prep Time: 20 minutes
Cooking Time: refrigerate for one hour or more

Here's a favorite dish for Thanksgiving or other holidays. I wanted to lower the use of refined sugar so I substituted the lovely flavor of maple with the richer flavors of brown sugar as opposed to white sugar.

½ cup maple syrup
1/3 cup brown sugar
1 pkg. cranberries
1 cup water

1. Place the water and sweeteners in a pot.
2. Cover and bring to a boil.
3. Add cranberries and cook over medium heat until all the cranberries have popped open to form a sauce.
4. Let cool. Pour into bowl and chill in refrigerator for at least one hour.

Serving Size and suggestions: Serves 8

Mashed Sweet Potatoes and Parsnips

Prep Time: 25 minutes

One year, I was tired of making plain mashed potatoes and candied yams for Thanksgiving dinner. I thought of mixing the two ideas together and came up with this recipe.

1 medium parsnip
1 medium-large sweet potato
1/8 - ¼ cup maple syrup
¼ cup soymilk, if desired

1. Scrub potato and parsnip with vegetable brush until clean. Cut into large pieces.
2. Place parsnip and potato pieces into large pot.
3. Fill pot with 4 cups of water. Bring water to a boil.
4. Lower to medium heat, to keep water simmering. Cook for about 15 minutes.
5. When vegetables are able to be easily pierced with a fork, remove from heat and drain.
6. Put vegetables into a large bowl, mash with potato masher.
7. Add maple syrup, and if necessary soymilk, and mash thoroughly until creamy.

Serving Size and suggestions: Serves 4-6, depending on size of meal.

Baked Acorn Squash

Prep Time: 15 minutes
Cooking Time: 1 hour

This is a recipe my mom used to make for Thanksgiving when I was a girl. It is still one of my favorites.

3 medium acorn squash
6 tsp. butter
6 tsp. pure maple syrup
water

1. Preheat oven to 375°.
2. Cut squash in half and remove seeds.
3. Make several deep cuts in squash from inside, being careful not to cut through the skin.
4. Fill baking dish with ½' of water. Place squash, skin side down, in water.
5. Put 2 tsp. each of butter and maple syrup in each squash half.
6. Cover each piece tightly with foil and bake for one hour.

Serving Size and suggestions: Serves 6.

Variations: Some people like to add a sprinkle of cinnamon or nutmeg to this recipe.

Holiday Date Bars

Prep Time: 15 minutes
Cooking Time: 25-30 minutes

This recipe was inspired by memories of my Mother's Joy of Cooking Date Bars *she made for us as kids. I prefer the natural sweetness of the dates without the graininess of granulated sugar. This version uses a little maple syrup instead and for some, is still too sweet.*

¾ cup maple syrup
1 ½ cups whole wheat pastry flour
3 eggs
1 ½ tsp. baking powder
1 tsp. vanilla
1/8 tsp. seasalt
2 cups chopped dates

1. Chop dates or purchase pre-chopped packaged dates.
2. Measure and then sift the flour, seasalt and baking powder.
3. Beat the eggs and maple syrup until frothy.
4. Mix the liquids with the sifted ingredients.
5. Add vanilla and dates and mix well.
6. Pour batter into lightly greased 9" x 13" pan.
7. Bake at 325° for 25-30 minutes.

Serving Size and suggestions: Makes 12-15 large bars. Delicious served with vanilla rice dream to drink or the frozen non-dairy ice creams.

Variations: Add ½ cup walnuts for a crunchy version.

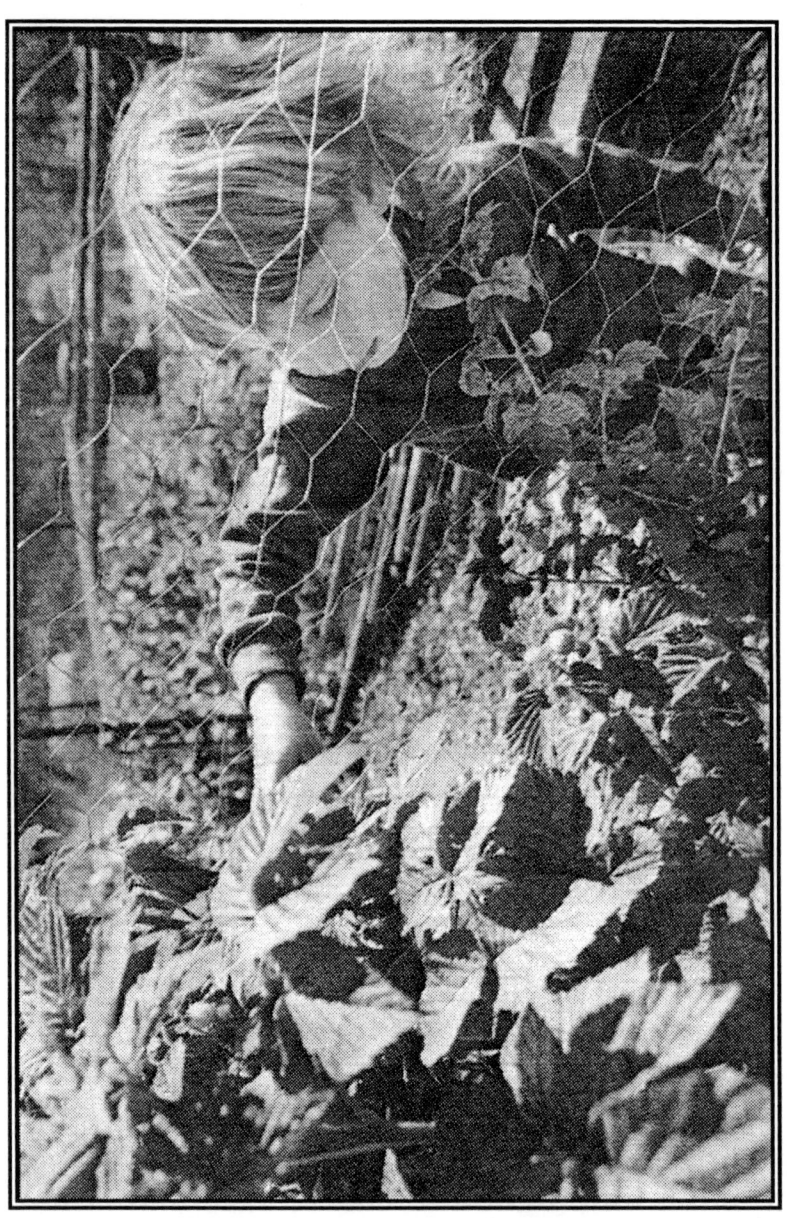

✧✧✧✧✧✧✧

"When sugar is used in moderation, it can prove to be a good medicine. It is unfortunate that modern man overuses it for purposes other than medicine or even simple satisfaction."
Naboru Muramoto

✧✧✧✧✧✧✧

Delicious Desserts and Drinks

Lemon Mousse Pudding

Prep Time: 10-15 minutes
Cooking Time: no cooking needed; refrigerate overnight before eating

This dish was created when I was craving a yummy, rich pudding for dessert. I loved pudding as a girl and have spent hours trying dairy-free alternatives. Finally I found that tofu is a perfect secret ingredient, not soymilk which was always too runny and not creamy enough. I thank Mori-Nu silken tofu for their inspiring product that made my dreams come true!

4 Tbsp. fresh lemon juice
¼ cup brown rice syrup
1 box Mori-nu silken tofu, firm
½ tsp. lemon zest
¼ cup pure maple syrup
1 tsp. vanilla

1. Place all ingredients in a blender and blend until smooth. I like to use my hand-held cuisinart for this instead. It's quick and easy.
2. Fill serving dishes with pudding and refrigerate overnight.
3. Lick the dishes clean before you wash them!

Serving Size and suggestions: This makes about 6, ¼ -½ cup servings. Excellent in summer garnished with red raspberries and a thin slice of lemon.

Banana Pudding or Pie Filling

Prep Time: 10 minutes
Cooking Time: refrigerate overnight

This pudding is a great guilt-free dessert. The pudding has a darker coloring on top when it sets, similar to the cream topping on some yogurts. This is not indicative of a spoiled pudding. It is a natural response of the banana's color change when ripe.

12.5 oz. silken tofu
1 ½ tsp. vanilla
1 ½ ripe bananas
¼ cup brown rice syrup
1 ½ Tbsp. maple syrup

1. Blend all ingredients until smooth and creamy.
2. Pour into individual serving dishes and refrigerate overnight.
3. Add sliced fresh banana to individual servings.

Serving Size and suggestions: Serves 6. Delicious served with vanilla wafers.

Nana's Noodle Pudding

Prep Time: 30 minutes
Cooking Time: 30 minutes

This is a recipe of my grandmother's, Nana. Every time she would visit she would make this dish for us. I made a few changes to make it fit my preferences, but the flavor is still true. (I left out the sugar, lowered the butter and added some soymilk.) It is filled with sour cream and eggs, so I only prepare it on occasion to fill my desire for a rich, nostalgic dish.

7 oz. egg noodles
3 small eggs
¼ tsp. salt
¼ cup butter
1 tsp. vanilla
1 cup sour cream
¼ cup soymilk

1. Preheat oven to 350°.
2. Cook noodles and salt in boiling water for 10 minutes, drain water.
3. Beat eggs until foamy, add soymilk, sour cream, butter and vanilla.
4. Mix noodles into egg mixture.
5. Grease 9x11" baking dish.
6. Pour noodle pudding into baking dish and bake for 30 minutes.

Serving Size and suggestions: Serves 6.

Variations: For a sweeter version, add ¼ cup of honey and ½ cup of raisins with a dash of cinnamon.

❧❧❧❧❧❧❧❧❧

Carob Brownies with Pudding Top

Prep Time: 20 minutes
Cooking Time: 25 minutes, refrigerate 30 minutes

I love desserts! I decided it was time for a brownie that was deserving of the name. This is moist with a "can't get enough of it" pudding on top. Indulge yourself, guilt-free.

½ cup butter (or margarine for dairy-free)
2 eggs
1 Tbsp. water
1 cup whole wheat pastry flour
¼ cup carob powder
½ cup pure maple syrup
1 tsp. pure vanilla
1 tsp. baking powder
¼ tsp. seasalt

Pudding:
¼ cup + 1 Tbsp. carob powder
10.5 oz. Mori-nu silken tofu, firm
¼ cup brown rice syrup
1 tsp. pure vanilla
¼ cup pure maple syrup

1. Preheat oven to 350°.
2. Melt butter.

3. Beat together butter, carob powder, maple syrup, eggs, water and vanilla.
4. Sift flour, salt and baking powder into carob mix.
5. Stir until mixed well.
6. Grease 8" square pan.
7. Pour batter into greased pan and bake for 20-25 minutes.
8. Remove from oven and cool.
9. Blend all pudding ingredients until smooth and creamy.
10. Generously spread pudding on cooled brownies.
11. Refrigerate 20-30 minutes, if desired.

Serving Size and suggestions: Serves 12-16. Top with frozen vanilla ice dream for a special treat!

The pudding can be made as a dish all on it's own. Prepare as in number 8 and pour into individual serving dishes. Refrigerate for one hour and serve.

Crispy Rice Bars

Prep Time: 10 minutes
Refrigerate overnight

I have a sweet tooth that has been hard to beat. In order to "have my cake and eat it too" I have created a number of scrumptious, sweet desserts that do not have any refined sugar in them. This recipe was inspired by my memories of those sickeningly sweet rice krispy bars from childhood. This is a much tastier and healthier version!

¾ cup brown rice syrup
3 cups crispy brown rice cereal (Erewhon)
1 Tbsp. barley malt syrup
¾ cup chocolate chips (barley malt sweetened) or carob chips
canola oil

1. Melt brown rice syrup and barley malt in a small pot until it is easily poured.
2. In a large bowl, pour the rice cereal and the chocolate chips.
3. Grease a 8x8 square baking pan with the canola oil.
4. Pour the melted syrups into the cereal and stir quickly until the cereal is well coated.
5. Pour the cereal mixture into the baking pan and refrigerate overnight. Cover bars with a glass lid or use plastic wrap for protection.

Serving Size and suggestions: Makes about 10-12 bars. These become quite gooey when warm, so they are best kept refrigerated up until it's time to enjoy them.

Variations: Leave out the chocolate chips for a chocolate-free version or use carob chips instead!

꙳꙳꙳꙳꙳꙳꙳꙳

Nut Butter Cookies

Prep Time: 20 minutes
Cooking Time: 8-10 minutes per batch

A delicious version of peanut butter cookies with the added twist of almond and no white sugar!

- 1 ½ cups peanut butter
- 1 ½ cups almond butter
- 1 cup brown rice syrup
- 3 tsp. vanilla
- 1 cup maple syrup
- 12 oz. malt-sweetened chocolate chips
- 4 tsp. baking powder
- 1 tsp. seasalt
- 1 cup unbleached white flour
- 2 ½ cups whole wheat pastry flour

1. Preheat oven to 350°.
2. Mix nut butters, vanilla and sweeteners thoroughly.
3. Add chocolate chips to mixed ingredients and stir well.
4. Add dry ingredients and be sure all of them are completely mixed in.
5. Form into cookies on baking sheet.
6. Bake for 8-10 minutes or until lightly browned around the edges.

Serving Size and suggestions: Makes about 60, 2" cookies.

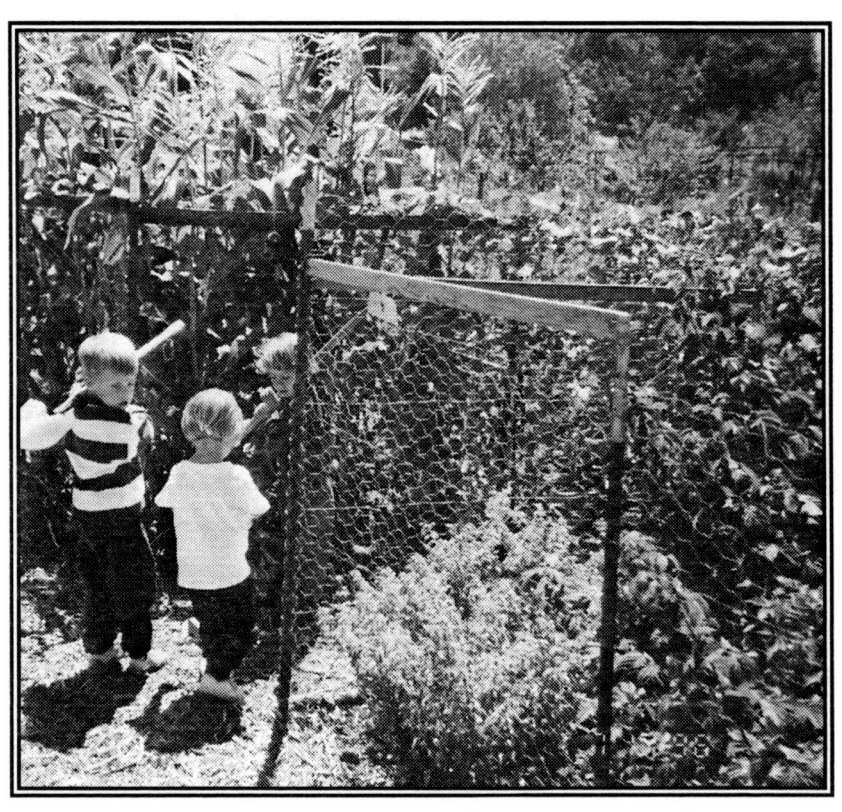

Ofer's Chocolate Cookies

Prep Time: 15 minutes
Cooking Time: 8 minutes per batch

My husband created these cookies when we were looking for a homemade version of some cookies we had from a health food store. Knowing that fresh is even better, Ofer came up with this recipe and they are to die for! For the true chocoholic. These cookies are wheat-free.

½ cup butter, very soft or melted
2 eggs
2 Tbsp. water
½ cup tapioca flour
2 cups brown rice flour
¼ cup molasses
1/3 cup honey
¼ cup cocoa powder
½ Tbsp. vanilla extract
½ tsp. baking powder
½ tsp. seasalt
1 cup chocolate chips
½ cup yogurt chunks

1. Preheat oven to 300°.
2. Mix dry ingredients in a large bowl.
3. With mixer, blend eggs, molasses, honey, vanilla, water and butter in a small bowl.

4. Pour wet ingredients into dry ingredients and stir until thoroughly mixed.
5. Add yogurt chunks and chocolate chips and mix well.
6. Grease cookie sheet. Drop dough onto sheet.
7. Bake for 8 minutes or until golden brown.

Serving Size and suggestions: Makes 2 dozen cookies.

Peanut Butter Cups

Prep Time: 40 minutes
Cooking Time: overnight refrigeration

I don't know about you, but when fall comes my family starts thinking of all kinds of yummy holiday treats we can make! This recipe was an alternative to the overly sweet Reese's version. We couldn't resist the powdered sugar in it. Nothing else seemed to work as well. These are quite large when made in regular sized cupcake baking cups. For smaller ones, get the miniature cups. This makes a great holiday gift too.

1 cup smooth peanut butter,
¼ tsp. seasalt
¼ cup powdered sugar
1 ¼ cup chocolate chips, barley malt sweetened
¼ cup soymilk, more if needed

1. Melt 1 cup of chocolate chips in a small pan. Dribble half of soymilk in and mix as chocolate melts. Add more soymilk as needed to make chocolate smooth and glossy.
2. Use a spatula to fill the inside of the baking cups thoroughly.
3. Refrigerate for ten minutes.
4. Meanwhile, mix peanut butter, sugar, salt, and extra chocolate chips.

5. Spoon mixture into cooled baking cups and return to refrigerator for ten minutes.
6. Cover with more melted chocolate, sealing top of cup so that peanut butter cannot be seen.
7. Return to the refrigerator to set overnight.

Serving Size and suggestions: Makes 6-8 regular-sized baking cups.

Variations: Use crunchy peanut butter, vary the types of chips on the inside: yogurt, white chocolate, butterscotch.

Honey Carrot Cake

Prep Time: 20 minutes
Cooking Time: 30 minutes

This is a favorite of my son's. The first time I made it he kept asking me to make it again. He didn't like the nuts in it so I am offering no nuts as an option. With the creamy frosting, this is a dessert as nutritious as a meal!

1 ½ cups whole wheat pastry flour
1 ½ cups unbleached flour
¼ cup canola oil
4 eggs
1 cup honey
½ cup brown rice syrup
2 - 2 ½ cups grated carrots
½ cup applesauce
½ tsp. seasalt
½ tsp. baking soda
1 Tbsp. baking powder
½ tsp. cinnamon
½ tsp. ginger
1 tsp. vanilla
1 cup walnuts, optional

1. Pre heat oven to 350°.
2. Oil a 10x13" pan.
3. Grate carrots.

4. Put honey and brown rice syrup in a small pot over low heat.
5. Sift flours, seasalt, baking soda and powder into a large bowl.
6. Blend melted sweeteners, oil, and vanilla.
7. Add applesauce and spices.
8. Mix well.
9. Pour wet ingredients into dry ingredients and mix thoroughly.
10. Add carrots and walnuts, if desired. Mix well.
11. Blend eggs for 10 minutes and fold gently into batter.
12. Pour into oiled baking pan and bake for 30 minutes.

Serving Size and suggestions: Makes a large cake, 24 pieces 2"x2". Delicious topped with Creamy Frosting (page 207, double recipe for 10x13 cake). Also great plain.

❧❧❧❧❧❧❧❧❧

Strawberry-Nutella Ladies

Prep Time: one hour, refrigerate for three hour before serving

My husband and son are especially fond of a wonderful spread called Nutella. It is made of cocoa and hazelnut. I was looking for a way to use the jar I had had in my cupboard for months and this lovely recipe is the result! I used the ladyfingers as a throwback to my childhood and they're still delicious.

1 pkg. (24) ladyfingers
2 Tbsp. lemon juice
4 Tbsp. Nutella + 3 Tbsp. water
1 pint strawberries
1 recipe Creamy Frosting (page 207) +
  2 oz. dairy-free cream cheese

1. Wash strawberries and remove stems.
2. Thoroughly blend 2 Tbsp. lemon juice with 6 strawberries to make a ½ cup of strawberry sauce.
3. Pour the strawberry sauce evenly over the bottom of an 8x8 pan.
4. Mix 4 Tbsp. of Nutella with 3 Tbsp. of water until the Nutella is of a spreadable consistency.
5. Place 10 of the ladyfingers with the rounded side down onto the strawberry sauce.
6. Spread the Nutella over the ladyfingers so it is evenly covering them.

7. Place 11 ladyfingers, flat side down on top of the Nutella spread.
8. Make the Creamy Frosting and add 2 oz. cream cheese and 6 strawberries.
9. Pour the frosting over the ladyfingers.
10. Slice the remaining strawberries and place in an attractive manner on top of frosting.
11. Chill for 3 or more hours before serving.

Serving Size and suggestions: Makes about 12, ½ cup servings.

Variations: Dip some strawberries in the Nutella spread and use them to decorate instead of plain strawberries.

Creamy Frosting

Prep Time: 10 minutes

This is a luscious topping for cakes or an excellent dip for fresh fruit. Decadent and simple, filled with healthy stuff.

- 8 oz. Tofutti cream cheese, plain
- 6 oz. firm silken tofu
- 1/3 cup honey
- ¼ cup brown rice syrup
- 1 tsp. vanilla
- 1 Tbsp. lemon juice

1. Put all ingredients in a bowl.
2. Blend until completely smooth and creamy, about 3 minutes.

Serving Size and suggestions: Double recipe for Honey Carrot Cake (page 203). To make a thicker frosting, add 4 oz. cream cheese. Serve on Carob Brownies with Pudding Top (page 193) instead of pudding top.

Vanilla Yogurt with Fruit and Carob Chips

Prep Time: 15 minutes

This is an elegant and simple dessert for summer banquets.

- 3 cups vanilla yogurt (your favorite brand, mine is Brown Cow with the cream on top)
- 2 large peaches
- 2 large bananas
- 1 small basket strawberries
- ½ -1 cup carob chips

1. Wash fruit and cut into bite-sized pieces.
2. Put yogurt into large bowl.
3. Mix fruit into yogurt.
4. Sprinkle top with ¼ - ½ cup carob chips. Serve extra carob chips on the side.

Serving Size and suggestions: Makes 6, ½ cup servings.

Variations: Instead of the fruit listed above, use a combination of berries: blackberries, red and yellow raspberries, strawberries and blueberries.

Lemon Tofu-Cheesecake

Prep Time: 40 minutes
Cooking Time: 2 hours until done

This dairy-free cheesecake is as rich and delicious as a traditional cheesecake. I love to eat this cake and feel that I'm getting my day's protein in at the same time!

Pie Crust: 2 Tbsp. soymilk
2-3 Tbsp. water, as needed
2 cups graham cracker crumbs
1 ½ Tbsp. melted butter or canola oil
1 Tbsp. brown rice syrup

Filling: 2/3 cup soymilk
2 ½' stick of agar
2 Tbsp. brown rice syrup
3 tsp. grated lemon rind
2 tsp. vanilla
¼ cup maple syrup
16 oz. silken tofu, firm
5 Tbsp. lemon juice
½ tsp. seasalt

Glaze: 1 Tbsp. maple syrup
½ tsp. grated lemon rind
1/3 cup brown rice syrup and honey, combined
2 Tbsp. lemon juice
¼ cup water
2 Tbsp. cornstarch

1. Crumble graham crackers by placing in a plastic bag and rolling over with rolling pin until well crushed and measuring 2 cups.
2. Mix ingredients and press firmly into 9" pie pan.
3. Soak agar in soymilk while baking crust.
4. Bake at 350° for 10 minutes and set aside to cool.
5. To prepare filling: In a small pot, heat soymilk and agar, maple syrup, seasalt and brown rice syrup for 10 minutes or until agar is melted.
6. Add the remaining filling ingredients to the heated liquids and blend until smooth.
7. Spread into the baked pie shell and refrigerate for ½ hour.
8. Make the glaze by mixing all of the ingredients in a small pot.
9. Place over medium-low heat and whisk until thickened, stirring constantly to avoid burning.
10. Smooth over top of cheesecake and chill for at least 1 ½ hours to set.

Serving Size and suggestions: one 9" pie.

Variations:
Cherry Cheescake: Mix a 15oz. can of unsweetened bing cherries with 2 Tbsp. maple syrup. Warm the cherries with their juice in a pot over med-low heat. Stir 2 Tbsp. cornstarch into 2 Tbsp. cold water. Stir into cherries. Stir continuously until sauce is thick. Allow sauce to cool thoroughly. Leave off steps 8-10 above, refrigerate cheesecake for 1 hour or until set. Spread thickened cherries over top and chill for another hour before serving.

Blackberry-Peach Cobbler

Prep Time: 20 minutes
Cooking Time: 30 minutes

At the local Farmer's Market, we get delicious organic fruit. One day, the vendors offered us 10 lbs. of bruised peaches and nectarines for a very good price. This cobbler was the best way I could think of to quickly use such a lovely offering.

2 c. blackberries
4 c. sliced peaches
3 Tbsp. lemon juice
1 Tbsp. brown sugar
¼ c. maple syrup
¼ c. unbleached white flour
½ tsp. cinnamon

Topping:
1 c. rolled oats
1 c. baby rolled oats
¼ c. unbleached white flour
1/8 c. raw wheat germ
4 Tbsp. butter, melted
¼ c. brown sugar
½ tsp. seasalt
½ tsp. cinnamon
1/8 c. minced almonds

1. Preheat oven to 375°.
2. Prepare fruit.
3. Mix brown sugar into maple syrup and pour over fruit.
4. Add lemon juice, cinnamon and flour. Mix well.
5. Pour into lightly oiled 8x8 baking pan.
6. Melt butter and mix topping ingredients with melted butter.
7. Spread topping over fruit and pat down lightly when evenly distributed.
8. Bake for 30 minutes.

Serving Size and suggestions: Makes about 9 good-sized servings. Delicious with vanilla ice cream like all cobblers are!

Variations: Leave out the berries for peach cobbler or use different berries (raspberries, boysenberries, blueberries).

Blackberry-Blueberry Vanilla "Sushi"

Prep: 30-40 minutes

This is my son's first real recipe. He created the idea, I came up with the best way to implement it. The ingredients are per his instructions. I think he did pretty well. If you don't like the "sushi" part, just have the berries topped with the vanilla sauce. Delectable! (Don't worry, there's no raw fish or seaweed in this dessert sushi.)

1 ¼ c. water (more for softer rice)
1 c. sushi rice
1 Tbsp. brown rice syrup (more to taste)
1 pint fresh blueberries
1 pint fresh blackberries
2 c. soymilk
1 ½ Tbsp. corn starch in 1 Tbsp. water
1/3 c. maple syrup
1 Tbsp. vanilla
garnish optional: fresh sprigs of mint

1. Cook rice with brown rice syrup and water according to package instructions. Cool thoroughly.
2. Wash berries.
3. In a bowl, mash together with a fork or potato masher: 2/3 c. blueberries and 2/3 c. blackberries. Blackberries will become fairly liquid and blueberries will still have some small pieces uncrushed.

4. Warm soymilk and maple syrup in a non-stick sauté pan.
5. Add cornstarch mixed in water. Stir slowly to thicken milk for 5-7 minutes over low heat.
6. When thickened, add vanilla and turn off heat.
7. Mix mashed berries with cooked rice.
8. Form rice into small cylindrical sushi-like shapes, two to each serving plate.
9. Spoon a moderate amount of vanilla sauce over the "sushi". Sprinkle leftover berries on top, a few of both kinds to create an attractive display. Garnish with a sprig of fresh mint, if desired.

Serving size and suggestions: Makes about 18 pieces, 9 servings.

Strawberry-Banana Sorbet

Prep Time: 10 minutes
Cooking Time: freeze overnight, 10 minutes to create sorbet

Ofer and I were experimenting with our Champion juicer to see if we could make ice cream. Instead we ended up with this and it was delicious and refreshing.

2 ripe bananas
1 cup strawberries, whole with greens off
½ tsp. vanilla
¼ cup apple juice
enough soymilk to make 3 cups in blender

1. Put all ingredients into blender.
2. Blend thoroughly.
3. Pour into shallow pan and put in freezer overnight.
4. Just before serving, put dessert through a Champion-style juicer to create sorbet texture.

Serving Size and suggestions: Makes 2, 1 ½ cup servings. Top with whipped cream.

Optional garnishes: diced strawberries, or a sprinkle of chopped, roasted almonds.

Lemon-ginger Tea

Prep Time: 5 minutes
Cooking Time: 10 minutes

This concoction is fairly common these days. Often it is found bottled with echinacea added to it. I like to have it with a dab of honey during cold and flu season, especially if I am feeling a little dragged out or have a sore throat.

 4 cups water
 3 - 1/8"slices of fresh ginger root
 1 lemon, juiced

1. Place all ingredients in a glass pot.
2. Bring to a boil.
3. Simmer for 10 minutes. Serve hot.

Serving Size and suggestions: Makes 4 cups.

❧❧❧❧❧❧❧❧

Honey Lemonade

Prep Time: 10 minutes
Cooking Time: refrigerate for 1 hour or add ice.

My family loves fresh lemonade in the summer! I created this healthier version when I had a friend who gave me bushels of lemons from her tree. I like to squeeze lots of lemon juice and freeze it in amounts that fit this recipe, so I can simply defrost, mix and serve. It makes a great project for kids, too!

1 ¼ cup fresh lemon juice
8 cups water
¾ cup honey

1. Juice lemons, being sure to remove all seeds and especially large pieces of pulp.
2. Pour 1 cup of the water into a small pot with the honey.
3. Heat over low heat until honey is completely melted and absorbed into the water.
4. Pour lemon juice into a pitcher.
5. Add honey water and the remaining 7 cups of water. Mix well.
6. Add ice or refrigerate to desired temperature.

Serving Size and suggestions: Makes 8 cups. Serve with a garnish of fresh lemon or a sprig of mint.

Simply Delicious Apple Cider

Prep Time: 2 minutes
Cooking Time: 20 minutes

There's nothing like hot apple cider on a cold winter evening. This is a favorite of my son's. He likes to make it himself!

  4 cups unfiltered organic apple juice
  2 sticks cinnamon

1. Pour apple juice into a pot.
2. Add cinnamon sticks.
3. Heat over medium-high until bubbling a little.
4. Turn to low.
5. Stirring occasionally, allow juice to cook for about 15 minutes.
6. Some of the juice will evaporate, leaving a delicious perfect apple cider.

Serving Size and suggestions: 3-4 servings depending on the size of your mugs. Delicious as a dessert and with whipped cream on top with a dash of chocolate or cinnamon.

Nut milk

Prep Time: 10 minutes

This is a tasty drink that can be served plain simply for enjoyment or used as a substitute for soymilk in recipes. When substituting be aware of the change in flavor that will result. Different nuts add different flavors and may not be good with some recipes.

1 ½ cups almonds, blanched
sprinkle of nutmeg or carob, optional
½ cup water, more as needed

1. Place nuts and water in blender.
2. Turn on to high speed.
3. When thoroughly blended, add water to get desired thickness.
4. Strain, if desired, for smoother texture.
5. Serve warm or cold with a sprinkle of nutmeg or carob.

Serving Size and suggestions: 1 cup

Footnotes

Chapter Two
1. "Low-fat isn't always best", *USA Weekend*, April 3-5, 1998
2. "Farms may have to follow pollution rules", *Contra Costa Times*, March 6, 1998
3. "Get it down pat: a little butter is healthy", *Contra Costa Times*, January 14, 1998
4. "Different fats may raise or lower risk of breast cancer", *Contra Costa Times*, January 12, 1998
5. "Low-fat isn't always best", *USA Weekend*, April 3-5, 1998

Chapter Three
1. "Animal study shows no use for menopause", *Contra Costa Times*, April 23, 1998
2. "Are common chemicals scrambling your hormones?", *USA Weekend*, February 13-15, 1998
3. ibid.
4. "Healthy spread on its way to U.S.", *Contra Costa Times*, July 22, 1998
5. ibid.

Chapter Five
1. "Report finds world gets richer, Earth gets sicker", *Contra Costa Times*, May 12, 1998
2. "Study: Airborne Pesticides a Real Risk", *Contra Costa Times*, August 20, 1998
3. "Inhaled Steroids May Stunt Growth", *Contra Costa Times*, August 15, 1998
4. "Pesticides and brain tumors in children", *Delicious!*, May 1998
5. "Children at risk from pesticides in food", *Contra Costa Times*, January 30, 1998
6. "Farms may have to follow pollution rules", *Contra Costa Times*, March 6, 1998
7. "Thousands leave homes during fire at fertilizer plant", *Contra Costa Times*, January 5, 1998

8. "Modern distribution systems seen as cause of food poisoning rise", *Contra Costa Times*, December 10, 1997
9. "Environmentalists seek pesticide control review", *Contra Costa Times,* December 28, 1997
10. "New rules on tainted fish start Thursday", *Contra Costa Times*, December 17, 1997
11. "Upgrades sought for food safety", *Contra Costa Times*, December 28, 1997
12. "EPA bans use of toxic herbicide Bromoxynil on genetically engineered cotton plants", *Contra Costa Times.*
13. "Water safety puzzle: chlorine byproduct is found…at levels associated with elevated miscarriage risk, but is 'fundamentally safe' ", *Contra Costa Times,* February 11, 1998
14. "Banana with a difference", Mark Mulcahy, *The Good Times,* January 1998
15. "Limiting toxins in fertilizer proposed", *Contra Costa Times,* January 9, 1998
16. "What you can't see in drinking water can hurt you", *Contra Costa Times,* January 17, 1999
17. "Are common chemicals scrambling your hormones?", *USA Weekend,* February 13-15, 1998
18. "Fish offer clues to chemical role in human sperm count decline", *Contra Costa Times,* January 29, 1998
19. "River pollution linked to sex defects in fish", *Contra Costa Times,* September 22, 1998

Chapter Six
1. "Trade rift over biotech food will force long-term studies", *Contra Costa Times,* July 14, 1999
2. J. Nordlee et al., "Identification of a Brazil-nut allergen in transgenic soybeans," *The New England Journal of Medicine* 334:688-92, 1996.
3. *Mothers for Natural Law, Consumer Right to Know campaign* 1998.
4. ibid.
5. ibid.

Recipe Index

Agar 209
Almond Butter 197
Appetizers -
  Stuffed Portabella Mushrooms 53
  Tofu-stuffed Wontons 55
Apple -
  juice 215, 218
  sauce 203
Artichoke - 49
  hearts 63
Asparagus 141
Avocado - 49, 50, 71, 86
  guacamole 51, 150
Bacon bits, vegetarian 113
Banana 190, 208
Beans -
  aduki 112
  black 75, 77
  black soy
  garbanzo 168
  kidney 83, 151, 175
  lentils 101
  navy 113
  pinto 175
  refried black 51
  refried pinto 51
  Aduki Beans with Kombu 112
  Barbecue Baked 113
Beets 81, 141
Bell Pepper -
  green 79, 125, 129, 139
  red 79, 129, 171
  yellow 53, 125

Berries -
  blackberries 208, 211, 213
  blueberries 208, 211, 213
  boysenberries 211
  cranberries 182
  raspberries 189, 208, 211
  strawberries 205, 208, 215
Bread -
  crumbs 53, 133, 168, 181
  pita 61, 71, 168
  sourdough 65
  whole wheat 50, 57, 181
  whole wheat sourdough 59
Broccoli - 96, 107, 122, 125, 139, 152, 159, 171
  Broccoli in Cheesy Sauce 179
Cabbage -
  green 79, 93, 97, 133
  red 79
Carob -
  chips 195, 208
  powder 193
Carrot 79, 93, 96, 97, 101, 103, 107, 122, 135, 139, 141, 145, 161, 165, 173, 203
Casseroles -
  Layered Enchilada 125
  Green Bean and Mushroom 127
  Corn 129
  Baked Eggplant Feta 131
  Baked Fish with Creamy Cabbage 133
  Stuffed Steamed Greens 135
  Stuffed Squash 137
  Roasted Winter Vegetables 139
  Red Veggie Surprise 141
  Mexican-style Pasta Casserole 149
Cauliflower 107, 122, 125, 139, 152, 171, 179

Celery 53, 89, 97, 101, 117, 181
Cereal, brown rice 195
Cheese -
  asiago 59, 65, 69, 70, 129, 131, 147, 151, 161
  cheddar 51, 57, 149, 161, 179
  feta 61, 71, 75, 86, 131
  monterey jack 59
  mozzarella 63, 65, 147, 149
  parmesan 53, 63, 69, 70, 131, 133, 147, 151, 153, 161
Cherries 210
Chocolate -
  chips 195, 197, 199, 201
Cocoa powder 199
Corn 77, 82, 83, 125, 129, 139, 149, 151, 159, 161
Cream Cheese 205, 207
Cucumber 86
Dates 185
Desserts -
  Carob Brownies with Pudding Top 154, 193
  Holiday Date Bars 185
  Lemon Mousse Pudding 189
  Banana Pudding or Pie Filling 190
  Nana's Noodle Pudding 191
  Crispy Rice Bars 195
  Nut Butter Cookies 197
  Ofer's Chocolate Cookies 199
  Peanut Butter Cups 201
  Honey Carrot Cake 203
  Strawberry-Nutella Ladies 205
  Creamy Frosting 207
  Lemon-Tofu Cheesecake 209
  Cherry Cheesecake 210
  Blackberry-Peach Cobbler 211
  Blackberry-Blueberry Vanilla "Sushi" 213
  Strawberry-Banana Sorbet 215

Dips -
  Avocado   49
  Layered Mexican   51
Drinks -
  Lemon-ginger Tea   216
  Honey Lemonade   217
  Simply Delicious Apple Cider   218
  Nut Milk   219
Edamame   82
Eggplant -
  globe   131, 147
  Japanese   75, 139
Eggs   129, 168, 185, 191, 193, 199, 203
Fish -
  swordfish   133
  tuna, canned   57, 85
  tuna, fresh   133
Flour -
  brown rice flour   199
  tapioca flour   199
  unbleached white   197, 203, 211
  whole wheat pastry   127, 157, 179, 185, 193, 197, 203
Ginger, fresh   55, 159, 173, 216
Graham Crackers   209
Grains -
  barley   93, 97
  bulgur   117, 119, 137
  couscous   117, 118, 141
  millet   118
  quinoa   118, 119
  rice, brown   107, 117, 121, 168
  rice, Japanese sushi   213
  Quinoa-Bulgur Pilaf   119, 135, 141
  Rice Pilaf   117, 135
  Simple Spanish Rice   121
Green beans   83, 107, 127, 139, 145, 165, 167

Greens -
  chard 107, 135, 161
  collards 107, 135, 137, 145
  kale 107, 137
  spinach 137, 149, 153
Herbs -
  basil, lemon 70, 82, 87, 145
  basil, sweet 69, 70, 96
  mint 75, 81, 82, 213
  parsley, curly 125, 165
  parsley, Italian 69, 75, 82, 96, 145
  savory 145, 165
Ladyfingers 205
Lemon Juice 49, 51, 55, 71, 79, 121, 189, 205, 207, 209, 211, 216, 217
Lime 75, 121
Miso -
  barley 57, 107, 122
  white 50, 85, 87, 103, 122
  red 85, 122
Mushrooms -
  crimini 161
  portabella 53, 59
  shiitake 59, 103, 161, 167, 173
  white button 63, 65, 107, 139, 153, 161, 181
Noodles, egg 191
Nutritional Yeast 129, 137, 157, 179
Nutella 205
Nuts -
  almonds 89, 141, 211, 219
  pine (piñon) 69, 117, 181
  walnut 70, 185, 203
Oats -
  baby rolled 211
  rolled 211

Oil -
  Chinese sesame 55, 103, 159, 165, 167, 169
  garlic 75, 96, 140, 147
  olive 53, 63, 65, 67, 69, 70, 71, 75, 82, 86, 93, 118, 119, 137, 139, 145, 151, 153, 161, 163, 175
Olives -
  black 51, 68, 125, 131, 149, 151
  green 65, 68, 86, 129, 139, 149
  kalamata 71, 139
Parsnips 107, 139, 141, 183
Pastas -
  bow 149
  fusilli 145
  lasagna 147
  macaroni 149
  vermicellli 153
  Amy's Anything Goes Garden 145
  Eggplant Parmesan Lasagna 147
  Mexican-style Pasta Casserole 149
  Multi-color 151
  Spinach Lasagna 147
  Spinach-Mushroom Pesto over Vermicelli 153
Peach - 208, 211
Peanut Butter 197, 201
Peas -
  fresh 82
  frozen 151
  snow 79
Pesto 59, 63, 65, 69, 70
Pickles 89
Pineapple -
  chunks 171
  juice 171
Pizza -
  Pesto Pizza 63
  Yummy Summer Sandwich Pizza 65

Potatoes -
  red 139
  russet 95, 99
  sweet 95, 105, 183
  yam 95
  yellow Finn 139
  Mashed Sweet Potatoes and Parsnips 183
Quiche 161
Radish -
  daikon 97
Raisins -
  black 191
  golden 79, 93
Salads -
  Black Bean with Mint, Lime and Herbs 75
  Black Bean, Corn and Tomato 77
  Colorful Coleslaw 79
  Cool Beet 81
  Fresh Peas with Edamame and Herbs 82
  Green Bean 83, 154
  Salat Tuna 85
  Israeli Cut Salad 85
  Sliced Tomatoes with Lemon-basil Miso Dressing 87
  Tempuna 89
Salsa 51, 121, 149
Sandwiches -
  Avocado-Miso 50
  Grilled Salat Tuna-Cheese 57
  Open-face Mushroom 59
  Pita with Roasted Vegetables 61
  Yummy Summer Sandwich Pizza 65
Sauces -
  barbecue
  marinara, mushroom and onion 67
  pesto 131, 153

pizza   131
  sweet and sour   55
  tahini   71
  teriyaki   163, 173
  tomato   67, 125, 149, 175
Sausage, vegetarian   137, 147, 149
Seaweed -
  kombu   103, 107, 112
  laver   103
  nori   103, 107
  wakame   97
Seeds -
  sesame   79, 141, 171
  sunflower   79, 119
Soups -
  Cabbage   93
  Creamy Squash and Potato   95
  Flame Carrot Dish   96
  Delicious Delicata Squash Barley   97
  Garlic   99
  Lentil Bean Carrot   101
  Seaweed   103
  Sweet Autumn   105
  Vegetable Rice   107
Sour Cream   51, 150, 191
Soy -
  beans, green (edamame)
  milk   79, 99, 105, 127, 133, 157, 179, 183, 191, 201, 209, 213, 215
  sauce (tamari)   59, 101, 112, 121, 135, 159, 165, 167, 169, 171, 173
  Black Soy Bean Sauté   159
Spinach   157, 161
Sprouts, mung bean   173

Squash, Summer -
  peter pan 65, 135
  yellow 63, 75, 135, 145, 165
  zucchini 63, 65, 75, 107, 125, 129, 135, 145, 161, 171
Squash, Winter -
  acorn 184
  butternut 95, 97, 105, 137
  delicata 97
  kabocha 95, 97
  Baked Acorn Squash 184
Stuffing 181
Sweeteners -
  barley malt syrup 195
  brown rice syrup 189, 190, 193, 195, 197, 203, 207, 209, 213
  brown sugar 87, 113, 182, 211
  honey 79, 81, 83, 171, 173, 191, 199, 203, 207, 217
  maple syrup 113, 182, 183, 184, 185, 189, 190, 193, 197, 209, 211, 213
  molasses 199
  powdered sugar 201
Tahina 57, 61, 71, 79, 85, 168
Tempeh 89,
  Barbeque Tempeh 164
  Early Summer Vegetables with Tempeh 165
  Green Bean Sauté with Tempeh and Shiitakes 167
  Tempelafel Patties 168
  Sesame Tempeh 169
Textured Vegetable Protein (TVP) - 101, 125, 149
  Sweet and Sour TVP Strips 171
  Teriyaki TVP and Vegetables 173
  TVP Chili 175
Tofu -
  regular, firm 159, 161, 163
  silken, firm 55, 89, 103, 147, 157, 189, 190, 193, 207, 209
  soft 49

Baked Tofu   163
Spinach Soufflé   157
Tomatoes -
  canned   67, 93, 151
  cherry   77, 82, 159, 161
  red   57, 59, 63, 71, 86, 101, 129, 137, 139, 168
  roma   87, 107, 145
  yellow pear   77, 82
Tortillas, corn   125
Vanilla   185, 189, 190, 191, 193, 197, 199, 203, 207, 209, 213, 215
Vegetarian chicken broth   93, 96, 99, 101, 107, 117, 118, 119, 135, 141, 181
Vinegar -
  apple cider   55, 81, 113
  balsamic   59, 139
  red wine   77, 82, 83, 85
  rice   55, 87, 171
Wheat Germ   211
Wine -
  cooking Sherry   53, 133, 173
  mirin   173
  red   59
Wonton   55
Yogurt -   79, 81, 208
  chunks   199